Medicine as Ministry

Medicine as Ministry

Reflections on Suffering, Ethics, and Hope

Margaret E. Mohrmann, M.D.

THE PILGRIM PRESS
Cleveland, Ohio

The Pilgrim Press, Cleveland, Ohio 44115
© 1995 by Margaret E. Mohrmann

Printed in the United States of America on
acid-free paper

00 99 98 97 96 95   5 4 3 2 1

Library of Congress Cataloging-in-Publication Data
Mohrmann, Margaret E., 1948–
Medicine as ministry : reflections on suffering, ethics, and hope /
Margaret E. Mohrmann.
p.   cm.
Includes bibliographical references and index.
ISBN 0–8298–1073–0 (alk. paper)
1. Medicine—Religious aspects—Christianity.   I. Title.
R725.56.M64   1995   95–18069
261.8'321—dc20   CIP

In memory of
SUSANNE HOGUE DEAS
Extraordinary and beloved friend
Struggling, shining witness
Mentor unaware

CONTENTS

❁

ACKNOWLEDGMENTS

❁

The major part of this book was originally prepared as a series of talks, presented in November 1991 at the annual conference "Medicine and Ministry of the Whole Person," at the Kanuga Conference Center in Hendersonville, North Carolina. I am grateful for the opportunity afforded by the invitation to speak there, and especially for the warm reception and thoughtful responses offered by the conference participants. Since 1978, I have attended many "Medicine and Ministry" meetings, invariably finding in them a community of love and respect, and of careful and passionate reflection on the tasks of healing as understood in the light of God. Therefore, my thanks are also for all the years of being embraced and taught by my friends there who demonstrate so much of what I speak of here.

Chapter 6 was first presented in May 1993 as the keynote address to a conference sponsored by the Roanoke Memorial Hospitals in Roanoke, Virginia. I thank the Rev. Richard Osmann, the hospitals' director of pastoral care, for asking me to speak, and thereby giving me the chance to formulate an approach to organ and tissue donation informed by theological ethics and by the themes of this book.

Several people have read and commented on my work at various stages. I am grateful for encouragement and suggestions from Jim Childress, Stan Hauerwas, Aline Kalbian, Cissy Lewis, Jane Lunn, Marty Perlmutter, Joyce Wooldridge, and my brother, the Rev. Ray Mohrmann. Roberta Culbertson was particularly helpful as a critical reader; she identified parts that needed to be thought through more carefully and expanded my understanding of many key concepts in the book. Deborah Smith's editorial suggestions have added significantly to the lucidity and coherence of these chapters. More important, she is a valued colleague and conversation partner in pediatrics who shares and enlarges my view of the meaning and privilege of our relationships with patients. Richard Brown, of The Pilgrim Press, has been as supportive and patient an editor as one could wish for.

I can only partially express, with these thanks, my appreciation for the overlapping circles of friends and colleagues who stimulate and foster my thinking and writing. Moreover, I remain ever indebted to the children and families who have been my patients. This book is an attempt to thank them for their generosity and trust, by telling what they have taught me, through their stories, about medicine's ministry.

INTRODUCTION

✳

This is a book about the conjunction of theological ethics and the practice of medicine. Consequently, it is a book about ministry, about service based on an approach to caring for the sick and suffering that is critically informed by the insights and imperatives of theology and theological ethics.

By identifying medicine as ministry, I am expanding the concept of medicine in terms of both definition and participation. Medicine as ministry is the work of caring for and promoting the healing of the sick and the suffering. In the ministry of medicine, health care professionals of various sorts are not the only ones who serve. We are all potential ministers of medicine within the healing community. In our homes, towns, churches, hospitals, and workplaces, we form moral communities with many tasks that need to be undertaken jointly, tasks like the rearing and education of our children and the relief of those among us who are poor. The work of medicine's ministry is also the responsibility of the community as a whole. Some members of the community, in their vocations as nurses and physicians and therapists, are indeed set aside specifically to be present with those who are ill, but we are all called to share in some way in that service.[1] To be complete, the healing community needs the participation not only of medical professionals, but also of lay ministers of healing, consolation, and presence, and of ordained ministers of healing, sacramental restoration, and blessing.

Therefore, throughout this book I speak of ministers, as well as physicians, in order to emphasize that most of what I have to say applies not just to medical doctors, nor even to hospital chaplains, but to all of us who in whatever fashion seek to serve those who are sick or in pain. I also refer to the one who suffers as the "patient." When I use this word, I speak of one who requires not only the help of a physician, but also the help of a pastor and of friends while undergoing the trials of pain and fear and fragile hope and inevitable change that illness and its treatment impose. The patient, in the context of this book, is anyone who is sick or in pain—physical or spiritual—to whom any one of us is called to minister.

By joining the ministry of medicine to theological ethics, I intentionally turn away from current methods and paradigms of standard biomedical ethics. There can be no question that biomedical ethics has added immeasurably to our understanding of what we are about in the doing of medicine. It calls the medical profession up short on its excesses and ignorances; it calls us to account for actions that can touch others' lives so deeply. It reminds us sharply about moral issues such as truth telling and can awaken us to the practical complexities of ethical principles like justice. However, I hold that biomedical ethics, as it is currently conceived and practiced, is an insufficient base for the sort of ethical ministry compelled by the suffering of those who seek medical care.

There are three areas in which the methods of biomedical ethics, when contrasted with the concerns of theological ethics, appear inadequate for supporting a broader concept of medicine understood as ministry: (1) the reliance of medical ethics on information that is insufficient and inappropriate for its moral conclusions; (2) its abstraction of unique stories into paradigmatic cases; and (3) its emphasis on seeking an answer (by implication, the "right" answer), on solving the problem.

To frame a critique of these three areas—a critique derived from the theologically based notion of medicine as ministry—consider the case of "Debbie." Debbie's situation was originally a startling story presented in the *Journal of the American Medical Association*; it is now a standard teaching case in medical ethics. A summary version of the case is as follows:

> A resident in gynecology is called late at night to see Debbie, a young woman whom the resident does not know. On reviewing her chart, the resident sees that she is in the terminal stages of ovarian cancer, wracked by pain and intractable vomiting. Entering her room, the resident notes her emaciated state and obviously great pain. Debbie mutters, "Let's get this over with." The resident calculates a heavy dose of morphine, knowing that it is necessary to relieve her pain but knowing also that it will surely cause respiratory depression and death.[2]

The question generally asked in reference to this case is, "Should the resident give the morphine?" This sounds like a reasonable question, given the situation, but in truth there is little or no moral information in the scenario that can support consideration of such a moral question. From the clinical information given, one can conclude only that Debbie is in the grip of inexorable suffering and is surely going to die, not what steps the doctor should now take.

Clinical information is a necessary background for moral deliberations about medical situations; the truth of Debbie's diagnosis and the severity of her pain matter crucially. But clinical information alone cannot lead us to moral conclusions. For moral conclusions, we need another sort of information in addition to the clinical. We need a knowledge of who Debbie is, what her life has been like, and what she wants her dying to be like. We need to know how her muttered statement fits or does not fit with how she has said she wishes to balance off those all-too-often conflicting goals of relieving pain and staying alive.

One can even say that the more interesting moral questions to be asked of this stripped-down story are: How could it happen that the last crucial question of Debbie's life is being asked of a resident she does not know, a doctor who knows nothing about her? How could it happen that the medicine practiced on Debbie and the medical education practiced on the resident could both be so lacking in ethical content as to leave the two of them facing each other in the darkness of her last morning without a moral leg to stand on?

Closely related to the problem of trying to reach moral conclusions without sufficient morally relevant information is the problem of abstraction. Debbie's case could as easily be about someone named Bill or Mary, dying of heart disease or AIDS or breast cancer; the real Debbie has already been abstracted out of the case. However, those who serve the suffering do not take care of abstract textbook figures whose problems are interchangeable. Patients are people who have names and faces; they have unique lives and unique deaths. To think that appropriate ethical answers can be found by abstracting those real persons out of their grounded, embodied, one-of-a-kind stories is to make a fundamental error in ethical reasoning.

There is a role for abstraction in medical ethics. At times, unfortunately, there are only abstract questions to be considered in making decisions on behalf of unconscious, unknown patients who appear to have no family or friends to speak for them. There are also abstract questions to be considered at the level of policy: criteria for admission to intensive care units, for decisions not to resuscitate certain patients, for retrieval of organs for donation from persons who are brain dead, for management of persons in a persistent vegetative state, for deciding who gets the available organs for transplant. All of these questions, and many other moral issues, require abstract discussions of our notions of justice and fairness, of how scarce resources are to be allocated, and of how we come to grips with definitions of personhood and of death. In contrast, the specific moral questions that affect the well-being of the real persons we know and care for are surely not best handled by treating those persons as though they were so many John and Jane Does, living generic lives, suffering generic afflictions, and dying generic deaths.

The third problem that I see with biomedical ethics, as it is commonly practiced and taught, is that its approaches can lead us to believe that we should seek the "right" answers to our moral dilemmas and, further, that such singular correct answers exist. Just as we can say with more or less assurance that Debbie's diagnosis and prognosis are accurate, we may think we can achieve comparable assurance and accuracy in answering the moral questions surrounding the end of her life. That is a dangerous illusion.

If we limit our understanding of the task in Debbie's case to seeking the "right" answer, we shall never break out of the impasse caused by the fact that, in her case as in so many others, there is more than one morally correct answer demanding our allegiance. There may be a broadly based consensus within medicine that the tasks of the physician are essentially to relieve suffering and to preserve life, but there is no consensus about which of these two goals is to take precedence when they come into conflict, as they do most poignantly in Debbie's situation. To search for an impossible "right" answer for how to minister to Debbie's urgent suffering is to risk moral paralysis, but to do nothing for her would be the most clearly wrong solution imaginable.

I suggest, then, that biomedical ethics is limited in its usefulness as a guide and model for the ministry of medicine because it deals with information that is inadequate to the task, it dwells too much in the abstract rather than with real patients within their complex and colorful lives, and it leads us to believe it is possible to find a correct answer to each of our moral questions. Theological eth-

7

ics, on the other hand, deals with a much broader and deeper understanding of the patient and of suffering, and with the need to remain focused on the particular afflicted person, in all his or her uncomfortable uniqueness. Theological ethics suggests that the best we can or should hope for from our moral ponderings is the fashioning of a way to act, a way to go on living, or a way of dying that fits a person's life—the careful and consensual fashioning of a fitting answer rather than the impossible search for the "right" answer.

Theological ethics is the study of the moral implications of theological statements and beliefs, of the way that God and our convictions about God do or should determine our character and our conduct, as individuals and as a society. What we believe about God critically forms what we believe about ourselves, our fellow human beings, and the lives we lead. Theological ethics, then, especially in relation to medicine, is not just about what should or should not be done in a particular instance. It is about how to understand what happens to us and what we do about it in the light of our existence as persons created to live and flourish within the universe embraced and sustained by God.

Theology—more specifically, Christian theology—is the framework for my ethical reflections on medicine understood as ministry. It is my intent to explore some basic Christian theological tenets to discern the implications they entail for our moral practice as ministers of medicine.

I begin with the belief that God is one, the basic monotheistic creed that illuminates and confounds our human tendency to turn many intrinsically good things—like health, and even life itself—into competing gods. I then consider the implications for medicine as ministry entailed by the Christian belief that the one God is also three, that the God in whose image we are created is understood to be a trinity, intrinsically and eternally relational.

The centrality of scripture is the next topic; I first examine its use as a moral resource. Then, an exploration of the narrative quality of scripture supports an approach to the care of suffering persons that acknowledges and honors the stories of their lives.

The resulting focus on patient narratives leads to a discussion of the metaphor of "writing the next chapter" as an alternative to problem solving. I explore the issue of organ donation, a frequently controversial area within biomedical ethics, in an extended interlude designed to highlight the theological approach to ethical questions in medicine and to exemplify a narrative understanding of the lives of those to whom we minister. Finally, I examine the sorts of rituals that enable and sustain a committed and compassionate ministry of medicine.

Throughout, my thesis is about the validity and utility of a broadly encompassing conception of medicine as ministry. Medicine, so conceived, is a service to those who suffer that draws its workers from within and beyond the ranks of medical professionals. This book is about how theologically formed ministers, whatever their jobs may be, can understand and practice the love God gives and expects within the arena of medicine, understood as ministry.

❀

CHAPTER I

GOD IS ONE

The Temptations of Idolatry

In 1979, the philosopher Alasdair MacIntyre wrote a provocative article in *The Journal of Medicine and Philosophy* titled "Theology, Ethics, and the Ethics of Medicine and Health Care." He began his essay with the following question and answer:

> What ought we to expect from contemporary theologians in the area of medical ethics? First—and without this everything else is uninteresting—we ought to expect a clear statement of what difference it makes to be a Jew or a Christian or a Moslem, rather than a secular thinker, in morality generally. Second . . . we need to hear a theological critique of secular morality and culture. Third, we want to be told what bearing what has been said under the first two headings has on the specific problems which arise for modern medicine.[1]

I shall not pretend that I am going to give a complete response to all that MacIntyre asks for in this passage. I do agree, however, with his insistence that any offering from theological ethics to the practice of medicine include statements of the unique theological bases of our ethical thought, criticisms of conventional culture, and the implications of theological beliefs and critiques for the sorts of issues that must be dealt with as we minister to those who suffer.

Let us start, then, with the premises that differentiate theological reflection from secular reflection—the premises that God exists, that God loves us, and that God is the Creator. One immediate corollary of the last statement is the understanding that, because God has created everything else, everything else is not God. We are, after all, monotheists, the coinheritors of the ancient Jewish revelation of the oneness of God. We are addressed in the Shema: "Hear, O Israel, the Lord our God, the Lord is One"; and we are disciplined by the commandment given at Sinai: "You shall have no other gods before me."

It is perhaps by now a cliché to say that, in our care for the suffering, we are assaulted, much like the Jews in the land of Canaan, by many temptations, many opportunities to put other, lesser, false gods before the one God. For example, it would be easy at this point to hold forth on the temptations of wealth for the physician. However, I shall not focus on this issue, because I think it is self-evident. No matter how bad physicians may be at acknowledging and combating the temptation of wealth, most of us are aware of it, at least at some level, and many of us even worry about it regularly. I doubt that I need to create discomfort about the queasy relationship between medicine and money.

It is another facile commonplace to bemoan our idolatry of medical technology and of those who know how to use it. Mother Teresa, for one, has called the neonatal intensive care units that populate American hospitals "obscene"; she could as easily have called them "blasphemous." But our adoration of machines and high-tech procedures is a superficial issue, and its elimination—even if that were possible—would still leave intact the deeper idolatry that supports it. The history of Israel shows us quite clearly that the destruction of the golden calf did not abolish idolatry from the hearts of the people of the covenant. Likewise, a wholesale attack on the worship of the icons of medicine will not eliminate the idolatry in our hearts that too often corrupts our use of those undeniably good inventions.

That idolatry within our hearts is more insidious and, I believe, far more worrisome than any enchantment by money or machinery. It takes two forms: the idolatry of health and the idolatry of life. The two are opposite faces of the same coin, both exhibiting the paradoxical mixture of pride and despair that characterizes the worship of false gods. David Barnard, in an essay on the relation of religion and medicine, has defined idolatry as "the denial of that wider context of meaning that endows the forms of worship with their sanctity."[2] I believe that both our idolatry of health and our idolatry of life manifest precisely such a denial of the wider context of meaning—the theological meaning—that alone gives health, and even life itself, whatever suggestion of sanctity either one may bear.

Reinhold Niebuhr has said that evil in its most developed form is always a good pretending or imagining itself to be better than it is.[3] The idolatry of health is a good example of this process, of pretending or imagining that the relative, subordinate good of health is better than God intends it to be. Evidence of the idolatry of health in our society is clear, manifesting itself in our fickle, shifting obsessions with diets and exercise machines and with jogging down every primrose path to perfect health, whether it is the path of vitamin C or brewer's yeast or no yeast at all or oat bran or whatever the latest "cure du jour." We have all been treated to, and have perhaps participated in, the spectacle of reasonable, pragmatic citizens of the last half of the twentieth century fearing and finding carcinogens everywhere, in much the same way our ancestors feared and found demons and witches everywhere.

It is also apparent that our idolatry of health goes hand in glove with an idolatry of the body, a presumption that health is entirely comprehended in physical health and, more particularly, in the physical health of a youthful body. Our single-minded focus on the health of the body is evident in the observation that even our interest in being mentally healthy—in handling stress, in expressing our feelings, in learning to be open and vulnerable—is often aimed at keeping us physically healthy. We try to be calm so we can avoid ulcers and heart attacks. We try to learn to laugh more so our arthritis will go away. We try to think positive thoughts so our immune systems will be stimulated to do their jobs more enthusiastically.

A true and complete understanding of health includes mental and spiritual health as important ingredients in their own right, not just as promoters of physical health. The biblical perspective on human life does not allow us to be dualists of the sort that denigrate the body as the prison of the spirit, but neither does it allow us to be dualists in the opposite sense, giving pride of place to the body and reducing our mental and spiritual faculties to mere maintainers and enhancers of our physical well-being.

What, then, are the implications of this situation for us who practice the ministry of medicine? What theological understanding of health can we bring to our ministry that can counteract and even redeem the idolatry that we find in our own hearts as well as in the hearts of those we serve?

First, we can bring to our work a balance and a perspective that come only from knowing that health can never be anything other than a secondary good. God is our absolute good; health is an instrumental, subordinate good, important only insofar as it enables us to be the joyful, whole persons God has created us to be and to perform the service to our neighbors that God calls us to perform. Any pursuit of personal health that subverts either of these obligations of joy and loving service is the pursuit of a false god. Health is to be sought in and for God, not instead of God.

Second, we must be aware of the extent to which the idolatry of health represents a failure of trust: trust, for example, in our own bodies to get us through life given a reasonable amount of care, trust in the food God provides and in those who supply it to us. It is certainly true that part of being good stewards of the bodies we have been given is to be careful. We need to recognize, for example, that there are practices in the food production system that can potentially endanger health, that there are some significant toxins floating around us, that there are ways in which our bodies break down despite reasonable care. However, such appropriate caution should be exercised in the context of a fundamental attitude of confidence that we have been created as far less fragile creatures than we fear we are.

A corollary to the belief that the God who loves us is the Creator is the belief that everything God has created is good. This does not mean that we cannot or do not contaminate what God has created. It means that we must not lose our basic theological assumption that our bodies and our food supply are to be trusted as good things, not feared as disasters waiting to happen. It is our task, as theologically formed ministers of health and healing, to witness to the goodness and the stability of God's creation, to be an antidote to the mistrust of creation manifested in obsessive searches for safe food and invulnerable bodies.

Even if we are not successful in transmitting our own faithful trust to those whom we serve, at least we can refuse to participate in that ignorance of God's creating goodness. For example, we can reject the assumption that normal children routinely need additional manufactured vitamins in order to be healthy, and the assumption that normal menopause is a "disorder" that routinely requires medical therapy, and even the assumption that a common symptom like the cough, God's brilliant mechanism for clearing the airways, routinely requires suppression whenever it occurs. Sometimes we are ridiculous.

Third, we must recognize the extent to which the idolatry of health represents a fear of death and often a denial of death's inevitability, both of which indicate a failure of hope. Several years ago, while browsing through a medical school library, I came upon a book titled *The Conquest of Death*, written in the mid-1960s. I examined it out of curiosity and found it to be a lengthy defense of the thesis that, given the pace of advances in medical knowledge and techniques, by the year 2000 no one will die except from catastrophic events like auto accidents and tornadoes. No one will die from disease or aging. There will be no "natural" death anymore.

The author was not very clear on whether our twenty-first-century immortality would also be accompanied by an arrest of the aging process. When I read the book, I found myself remembering the myth of Tithonus, the handsome hero loved by Eos, goddess of the dawn. She asked Zeus to grant him immortality, and Zeus did, but she had forgotten to ask also that he be given eternal youth. Poor Tithonus got older and older but could not die. Eos eventually had pity on him, after he had become so wizened that he had to be carried around in a basket, and turned him into a cicada. I thought the book was a pretty good joke—medicine as a producer of immortal crickets—until I started mentioning the book and its claim to groups of medical students. I found that at least half of them saw nothing odd in it at all and could not understand my reaction of amused disbelief. They really thought—and, I suspect, many of them still think—that eventually, by the grace of medicine, death will no longer be anything but an accident that befalls some but not most of us, and that we shall all coincidentally remain eternally twenty-five years old.

Odd books are not the only evidence of our fears and denials. The carelessness of the language we use in speaking of death reveals an underlying, and unexamined, assumption that at least some of us may be able to escape death. We speak of "preventing deaths" from cigarette smoking when we can only mean that people will then die, presumably at a more advanced age, for some reason unrelated to tobacco. We claim that people who fail to engage in certain health-promoting activities are generally "more likely to die," as though the general risk of dying could be anything less than 100 percent. These may not be intentional denials of the reality of death, but such linguistic slips betray a belief that drives the health-seeking behavior of many of us. It is the unspoken, but strong and pervasive, belief that if we just learn enough, do enough, prevent enough, exercise enough, eat the right stuff, purify our air and water and food, none of us will have to die.

We know better. We know that we are going to die. We know that death is the natural end to our earthly stories and even that it is to be welcomed as the mercy that it can be.

Some of us in the ministry of medicine do have the task of preventing untimely death, death that comes before the story has spun itself out; we rightly do this with all the medical know-how at our disposal. Others of us in the ministry of medicine have the task of preventing meaningless death, death that comes before the story has started to make sense; we do this by helping those we serve find some sense in the story. But none of us has the impossible task of preventing death. And all of us have the theological task of imparting hope—sometimes hope for an extension of earthly life, but always hope for life beyond death, in God.

We may not always be able to transmit our hope to those to whom we minister, but at least we can refuse to be part of the lie, part of the denial of the fact of death. That denial is an illusion that theology and theological ethics simply do not allow to enter into the ministry of medicine.

In Georges Bernanos's thoughtful and moving novel *The Diary of a Country Priest*, the priest's spiritual mentor tells him,

> Our Heavenly Father said mankind was the salt of the world, son, not the honey. And our poor world's rather like old man Job, stretched out in all his filth, covered with ulcers and sores. Salt stings in an open wound, but saves you from gangrene.[4]

Whether or not the salutary effects of salt on gangrene would bear scientific scrutiny, it is true that we are called to be salt and not honey. Moreover, we are all rather like Job, bearers of open wounds, one of which is often a dread of death that leads us to suppress our knowledge that it will happen. Part of our task as salt for the world is to sting that wound, to remind each other of something we would choose to forget, that Lazarus died again.

Many philosophers have said in various ways that it is the certainty of death that gives life its meaning. Flannery O'Connor expressed this idea in her own inimitable way in her short story "A Good Man Is Hard to Find." An escaped convict kills a foolish, garrulous, terrorized grandmother, just after she has granted him the touch of grace that is the hallmark of O'Connor's stories. He then says, "She would of been a good woman, if it had been somebody there to shoot her every minute of her life."[5] So would we all.

I do not suggest that we continually hold a gun to the heads of our patients, our parishioners, or our friends to remind them that they are going to die. We are talking about ministry, not about haranguing or terrorizing. But remembering that death will happen, that there is a limit to this life, changes the questions we ask of ourselves and of those to whom we minister. The question is not, "What can I do to live longer?" The question is, "How shall I live the life I have?" Health-seeking behavior is not death prevention; it is life enhancement. This change in attitude restores perspective and balance to our lives. It returns health to its proper, subordinate place as a means to living a joyful life of service, not as the goal in a death-denying search for immortal youth.

Along with the denial of death that drives the idolatry of health comes the other form of idolatry, the one to which I fear we of theological bent are particularly inclined. It is the idolatry of life, marked most distinctively by the all-too-frequent use of "sanctity of life" arguments in ethical discussions. Theologically speaking, there can be no argument based on a purported "sanctity of life," both because there is no "life" as such and because we are on very shaky ground when we speak of anything or anyone but God as unqualifiedly sacred. Let me explain what I mean.

When I was a youngster, my pastor once asked my church school class to find in the Bible the book of Hezekiah. It took all of us a few minutes of flipping through our Bibles to realize that there is no such book in the Bible; it simply *sounds* as though it should be there. I suspect you could play the same sort of trick on any number of people by asking them to find in the Bible the place where God says, "Let there be life." It sounds as though it should be there, but there is no such statement. God did not and does not create anything called "life." God created and creates living beings.

> Then God said, "Let the earth put forth vegetation: plants yielding seed, and fruit trees." . . . And God said,

"Let the waters bring forth swarms of living creatures and let birds fly above the earth.". . . And God said, "Let the earth bring forth living creatures of every kind.". . . Then God said, "Let us make humankind in our image." (Gen. 1:11, 20, 24, 26)

There is no life except as embodied in living beings, a truth we seem often to forget. Common enough to have become a standard caricature is the person who claims to love humankind but cannot stand people. Frighteningly common is the person who argues for sanctity of life while remaining oblivious to the plights of individual beloved beings who are the only forms in which that life exists.

When we, as persons who wish to live by a morality that is wholly theologically determined, are asked what we think about such issues as abortion, euthanasia, withholding hydration and nutrition from persons in the persistent vegetative state, or taking organs for transplant from anencephalic infants, the theologically appropriate response, the response of Christian ethics, is to ask in return, "To whom are you referring?" How can such issues even be addressed if we do not know whom they are about, or why they are being raised, or how the conclusions may be used?

Who is considering abortion and why? What is this person's story? Who is in a persistent vegetative state and what are the family members saying and doing? The policies and laws we help create must leave room for these queries. They must also ensure that the responses can be brought to bear on the decision in thoughtful, compassionate, and nondiscriminatory ways that consider the particulars of the situation without lapsing into reliance on the fraudulence of relative desert and worthiness.

The reply to the impersonal and empty claim of the sanctity of life, then, is always first the question, "Whose life?" Christian ethics is personal. As Dietrich Bonhoeffer wrote,

> Christ teaches no abstract ethics. . . . Christ did not, like a moralist, love a theory of good, but he loved the real man. He was not, like a philosopher, interested in the "universally valid," but rather in that which is of help to the real, concrete human being.[6]

What I am claiming, along with Bonhoeffer, about the Christian ethical focus on concrete persons in concrete circumstances may be met with the objection that this smacks of "situation ethics," and the Christian church, as a whole, has come out rather forcefully against situation ethics. In fact, in Christian circles, the term "situation ethics" is about as certain a conversation stopper and argument clincher as the phrase "secular humanism." No Christian wants to be thought of as supporting either one; each is considered to be clearly defined and as clearly rejected by both parties in any Christian dialogue. While I cannot speak for the definition and use of "secular humanism" as the knockout punch in any controversy, similar use of the label "situation ethics" is usually based on a misunderstanding of the term.

Joseph Fletcher's book *Situation Ethics*,[7] when it appeared in 1966, was roundly and rightly criticized by many segments of the church for the moral instability caused by its elimination of consistent anchors for moral decision making. Fletcher's argument, located explicitly within Christian ethics, is that the moral person does whatever love requires in the situation. Such a claim sounds unexceptionable until one realizes that he provides no significant structure for the discernment of what love does require. Fletcher has no reliable, consistent, historically and biblically grounded conception of what "Christian" love might mean. All the rules that Christians customarily consider to be at least partial and paradigmatic explanations of the way Christian love usually acts are reduced by Fletcher to mere guidelines, rules of thumb that can be discarded at will if the situation seems to demand it.

In contrast, the major strands of Christian moral thought through the centuries have insisted that the precepts found in scripture and traditionally promulgated by the church are not just guidelines for behavior but are, in fact, prima facie rules. That they are prima facie rules means that they can be overridden, that they are not absolute. There is no absolute in Christian ethics except the call to love God and love each other. However, prima facie rules, those paradigms we have been given of how love acts, cannot be simply discarded as the fancy strikes us, without a second thought. We can override them only in the service of another, equally compelling rule, and we cannot override them at all without experiencing and confessing the pain of doing so, the pain of recognizing our own sinfulness, the imperfection that makes such dreadful choices inescapable.

A true "situation ethicist" of Fletcher's sort would be able to say that love requires that the gynecology resident I mentioned in the Introduction relieve Debbie's suffering by whatever means necessary and that, given the terminal nature of her illness, the rule against killing need not be considered in her case. Alternatively, such an ethicist could say that love requires that the resident preserve Debbie's life at all costs, and that the precept about relieving suffering does not apply because it cannot be done in this case without also killing her.

We know it is not that simple, not that painless. Christian ethics insists that, whatever action is taken in Debbie's case, love requires mourning for the rule that cannot be followed. That the doctor cannot both preserve Debbie's life and relieve her suffering is the truth of the situation, but this does not mean that the commands to do both no longer apply. It only means that the doctor must violate one to accomplish the other, and that the doctor must mourn and repent that violation even while performing an act that is truly one of moral Christian love. This is what it means to be fallen people. Flannery O'Connor has written that "there is nothing harder or less sentimental than Christian realism,"[8] and Christian realism, like Christian love, demands that we acknowledge that real situations, involving God's real children, often require difficult and painful choices of us. They even require us at times, in the service of those we are called to love, to violate the very precepts that we hold most dear.

The "situation ethics" that Christianity has rejected has no place for that pain, no place for the residua of a decision to choose one precept over another when both apply, no place for the recognition of our inescapable sinfulness. It is its false clarity in the face of the ineluctable ambiguity of human dilemmas that makes "situation ethics" morally and theologically unacceptable, not its use of the details of the situation in reaching its decision.

Christian ethics has always required attention to the details of the situation. Despite Jesus' explicit acknowledgment of the importance of the law, he did not take up a rule, such as "Thou shalt not steal," and apply it as though it were a blind bludgeon, heedless of the circumstances. Consider his treatment of the thief Zacchaeus whom he loved into restitution; or of the thief Judas whose theft

27

from the common purse Jesus seems to have ignored in his persistent attempts to have his love penetrate Judas' misconceptions; or of the thieves who were money changers in the temple, whom he scourged; or of the thief who hung beside him on the cross, whom he forgave. These are all very different reactions to what some would call basically the same crime. They are all manifestations of divine love acting in the situation.

We always act within specific situations, and we must always be aware of and responsive to the details of those situations; the circumstances must be a vital part of what forms our moral decisions. In that sense, Christian ethics is very much situation ethics; it is not, however, the sort of rootless, painless, unrealistic situation ethics that Fletcher preached.

> Now there was a woman who had been suffering from a hemorrhage for twelve years; and though she had spent all she had on physicians, no one could cure her. She came up behind him and touched the fringe of his clothes; and immediately her hemorrhage stopped. Then Jesus asked, "Who touched me?" . . . When the woman saw that she could not remain hidden, she came trembling; and falling down before him, she declared in the presence of all the people why she had touched him, and how she had been immediately healed. He said to her, "Daughter, your faith has made you well; go in peace." (Luke 8:43–45, 47–48)

Jesus surely had the power to heal anonymously, but he chose not to. He insisted upon making that magical healing his own, accomplished on his own terms. He insisted also upon making the healing her very own, the healing of his particular daughter whose particular faith, and not some undirected magical power located in the fringe of his robe, had brought her into contact with divine healing love. We have no evidence that Jesus ever healed in any other way. When he fed the five thousand with loaves and fishes, he also had the power to award them a sort of blanket healing for whatever physical ailments they happened to bring with them that day, but he did not do so. To argue that he should have would be to misread both the nature of his power and the meaning of the incarnation.

The woman with the hemorrhage was healed before Jesus knew who she was, but he would not have it remain so. He would not be a party to magical, faceless healing. So it must be with us. "Who is this?" is always the question that must be asked by us if we are to evoke and enable the sort of healing love that God has manifested to us in Jesus. When the questions arise that attempt to put the biggest dilemmas of living and dying in terms of populations or generic categories or abstract descriptors—such as persistent vegetative state or unwanted pregnancy or Alzheimer's disease—the Christian is obligated to speak Jesus' words, and thereby to do what Karl Barth insists all

29

Christian ethics does: to repeat the good that has been said.[9] We are to say, "Who touched me?"

In the earliest days of Christianity, a common pagan objection to the idea of Jesus as the Christ was what is termed the "scandal of particularity." The "scandal" is the outrageous idea that God would become incarnate in one particular human being, subject to all the vicissitudes of a truly human, individual life. Although we know that our faith and our redemption are founded on the truth of that very particular incarnation, we keep repeating the pagans' mistake by refusing to accept the fact that the scandal of particularity continues, that such outrageous behavior is part of the essence of the nature of God. Christians do not believe that God is somehow generically present in something called "life." We believe that God is present in individual human persons. It is those persons whom we are called upon to love and serve, to respect and even revere in all their difficult and scandalous particularity.

Jesus does not call me to love the Ground of Being and to love life wherever I find it as much as I love the life force within me. I am, rather, called to love the very distinctive, singular, personal God of Abraham, Sarah, Deborah, and David, and to love the unique, imperfect, redeemed person who is my neighbor—just as I am to love the equally unique, sinful, and redeemed person who is myself.

Albert Schweitzer's guiding ethical principle of "reverence for life" is often cited as an important resource for our contemporary emphasis on sanctity of life. Although Schweitzer's own life and deeds of love are undoubtedly worth emulating, his ethical reasoning presents at least two insurmountable problems. The first, and perhaps most obvious, is that Schweitzer's formulation cannot serve as a basis for deriving any sort of human right to life. He extended his mystical principle to include all forms of living beings equally and thereby made problematic any higher value for human life, any way of consistently preferring to preserve the life of a human being rather than that of, say, a tapeworm.

The other, more important, problem with Schweitzer's principle is that it is unacceptable for any theological ethic.[10] For Schweitzer, life is the supreme good; life is the foundation and standard of all ethics, the highest and only lawgiver. In short, in Schweitzer's reasoning, life usurps the place of God. This is exactly the idolatrous danger we encounter when we fall into the habit of regarding physiological life as sacrosanct. This practice is called "vitalism"; it is idolatry.

Scripture is clear and consistent: God alone is sacred. That we are created bearing the image of God does not mean that we, too, are sacred beings. The sort of reverence we owe to the lives of human beings—including our own lives—is never absolute. God alone is holy. The church's traditional esteem for martyrs and scriptural warrants for believing that there are things worth dying for make no sense if human life is to have absolute value. Christian teaching affirms respect for every human being but it does not assume an infinite value for human life.

We may refer to human life as "sacred" only if we also admit the qualifications that only God is holy and that any holiness that can be attributed to any human being is derived from God's holiness. Our derived and conditional "holiness" is a function of our having been created by God, of our having been marked with God's image, and of our being loved and redeemed by God. As Reinhold Niebuhr put it, the command to love our neighbor is not based on the fact that our neighbor is equally divine or even that our neighbor is a person, but simply on the fact that our neighbor is beloved by God.[11] This is the source of the respect, and even awe, that we owe to every human being, and God's love, the source of our worth, is not given to us as faceless outcroppings of some generic life force.

The "sanctity of life" claim is unacceptable because it is impersonal and empty. It is an impersonal claim because the word "life" has no meaning except in the context of its embodiment in a particular person. It is an empty claim because our relative "sanctity" does not automatically tell us anything about what is to be done. "Sanctity" can be neither a synonym for "keep alive at all costs" nor, on the other hand, a code word for the sort of misguided compassion that assumes that the proper way to eliminate suffering is to eliminate the sufferer. "Sanctity" can only mean "beloved by God," and the God who loves us calls us by name.

God loves us as individual persons with unique characteristics, with hairs that can be numbered. This is how we are called to love one another—never as "sacred life," but always as beloved and particular living beings, with different needs, different problems, different stories. Because our stories, like our names, are different, honoring my life may require something very different from honoring your life, or Debbie's life.

When the time comes that I am suffering, or dying, or in an irreversible coma, and there are difficult decisions to be made on my behalf, I do not want those who care for me to talk about the "sanctity of life" as though the phrase has meaning. I want them to say instead, "Here is God's beloved, Margaret. How would God have us love her here and now?" I want them to look at me the way God looks at me. I want them to remember who I am, the themes of thought and action that have run through my life, and to make decisions for me that are congruent with the whole of my life as I have lived it. Christian ethics is personal; it is within that personal context that we must accomplish our tasks of ministry and healing.

❖

CHAPTER 2

GOD IS THREE
Metaphors of Relation

In the preceding chapter, the emphasis on the forms of idolatry that can be found within the ministry of medicine arose from ethical reflection on the theological belief in the unity of God, in God's absolute oneness. However, the God we worship and serve, the God revealed to us through Jesus, is not only one; God is three. Christians are trinitarian as well as monotheistic. I want now to point out what is important to our understanding of ourselves as the people of such a God in relation to our task of serving the suffering.

There are some unavoidable problems with the predominant metaphor we use to explain the triune nature of God to ourselves. The metaphor that describes the Trinity as Father, Son, and Holy Spirit has solid scriptural warrants that cannot be set aside at will. However, like all metaphors, it both enhances and obstructs our understanding; it conceals as well as reveals. The barriers to comprehension are strengthened by the fact that we usually forget that this language about God—like all language about God—is indeed metaphorical. All that we can ever say about God can be only figurative speech, approaching but never attaining a full grasp of God's nature.

In the case of the Father-Son metaphor, the main barriers to understanding are occasioned by the metaphor's being both exclusively male (although at times the Holy Spirit is referred to as a neutral "It") and intrinsically hierarchical. No matter how much we talk about God as not having gender and about all three persons of the Trinity as coequal and coeternal, it is virtually impossible for us to say "Father and Son" without making any number of automatic associations that are both gendered and unequal in rank and in time. It is very difficult for our finite, language-determined minds to imagine a father-son relationship in which the father is not in some way to take precedence over the son, and certainly in which the father must not have existed before the son, not to mention how difficult it is to work any kind of feminine reference point into the metaphor.

We cannot discard the Father-Son metaphor entirely without denying what we believe to be both the incarnate male form of the Christ and Jesus' references to the

Father. We can, however, explore other, equally warranted metaphors. More important, we can look behind all the metaphors to grasp the significance of what they teach us about the nature of God.

The search for other metaphors to depict the idea of trinity has recurred periodically throughout the history of Christian theology, most recently among feminist theologians. In the early church, Augustine's *De Trinitate* was the most influential explanation of the doctrine of the Trinity. Augustine based his arguments and exegesis not on the Father-Son metaphor, but on two analogs he introduced to make the idea of a three-in-one nature intelligible to his readers. First, he used the trinity of memory, understanding, and will that we can be aware of in the workings of our own minds. Second, he described the trinity required by our belief that God is love: the trinity of lover, beloved, and love.

The metaphor of lover, beloved, and love teaches us the same vital truth about God that lies behind the Father-Son metaphor. We learn that one fundamental significance of the doctrine of the Trinity is the revelation that God's nature, the very essence of God, is relational.[1] God is not monolithic; God contains within God's very self the reciprocity essential for the existence of love. God cannot be love without having an object to love and without being loved by that object in return. Thus the mutuality of love is primally and eternally constitutive of God.

Jesus teaches us clearly what this mutuality of love means. He tells us that he has received all that the Father has, that he can do only what he sees the Father doing, and that everything and everyone he has received, including all the glory that has accompanied his ministry, he continuously gives back to the Father (John 16:15, 5:19, 3:35, 5:30, 12:44, 17:10). The essential and eternal nature of God, the God who is love, is perpetual self-giving and self-receiving. The Father and the Son are both eternally involved in this mutual exchange, eternally giving to and eternally receiving from each other. The love that flows back and forth constantly in this mutual giving and receiving, the love that is this mutuality, is the Holy Spirit of God.

It is in this Spirit that we have been created in God's image. Creation according to the divine likeness not only is a descriptor of human nature, but also has normative implications. As images of God, we are to love as God loves. We are not God; we cannot be love as God is, but we are called, and therefore we are able, to express love according to the definition found within the nature of God: love as total, mutual self-giving and self-receiving.

Furthermore, because we are images of God, our essential natures also are relational. We are not God; we cannot form within ourselves, as God does, the relations that affirm our natures. Rather, the relations that constitute our very selves are "external" ones, with others and with God. Each of these aspects of our having been created in the image of a trinitarian God has implications for the practice of the ministry of medicine.

The giving and receiving that go on within the essence of God are complete. As finite human creatures, we may not be able to comprehend, much less accomplish, such a process of utter, continuous self-emptying and refilling. However, if we are to live as God's images, we must discern what the features of a human translation of the totality of God's love might be. We can look to the Bible for clues.

Jesus tells us of the liberality of the vineyard owner who paid top wages even to those who worked only one hour, and of the widow who gave her mite although it was all she had. He tells us of the Samaritan who not only gave first aid to the man injured on the road, but also guaranteed payment for his care without first asking for an estimate or setting a limit; we are not told whether this good Samaritan was a wealthy man. What these and other exemplary figures teach us is that the giving that characterizes our love is to be generous beyond our imagining. It is to be a careless, trusting, open-handed and open-hearted liberality that does not stop to calculate the cost in the face of need.

We who minister to those who suffer are called to love them, and this means that we are to give ourselves—our knowledge, our time, our faith, our passion, our strength— without stint. We are called to give exuberantly and extravagantly; there is no stinginess, no holding back, in love's service. Does this mean that we are to spend all our time at the hospital, all our time visiting and ministering to the sick and the needy in our community? By no means. Those who suffer are not the only ones we are called to love. Our families, our friends, and our own selves also have compelling claims on our extravagant love. We are not God; we are finite human beings who live in time and who must be good stewards of that time. However, we may not accept the notion that, if we shower love and mercy on those who suffer, there will be little or none left for the others we love. Rather, our love is like the widow's cruse of oil whose level never changed, no matter how much she took from it.

Having said this, I must admit that there are many times when we find ourselves drained, when we feel that we literally have no more to give. Some of us—and I am one of them—often feel that we must shield ourselves from what seems to be the black hole of suffering humanity, constantly threatening to suck us into its maw, from which there is no hope of return.

There are two things to consider about the experience of being drained. First, it is easy to mistake fatigue for emptiness. The tasks of discerning what, when, and how to give and then giving are physically and mentally exhausting. We must be good stewards of our limited energy as well as of our finite time. But being too tired to keep giving is not the same as being empty; being drained of energy is not the same as being drained of love.

The second and more important point is that we may indeed be drained of love, that we may truly have nothing left to give. This happens when we have stopped receiving, when we have turned off or blocked the channels that pour into us the love that can keep us full no matter how much we expend. The blockage happens in any number of ways. Our allocation of time may not have left room for the re-creating moments we need to spend with God alone, the time in which we open ourselves directly to the gift of God's overflowing love, God's Holy Spirit. Or, for various reasons, we may have closed ourselves off from the filling love that comes to us from family and friends or from our own care for ourselves, often, again, as a result of an imbalance in our stewardship of time.

Even more relevant to the discussion of our ministry of medicine is the observation that we may close ourselves off from the filling gifts that come from the suffering people whom we serve. Replenishing the self we pour out each day in love and service is not exactly like filling a car's gas tank. It is not so much that we expend the love in one place—in the office, the hospital, the nursing home—and then go somewhere else—home, a friend's house, a quiet place for prayer—to get refilled. Rather, the love that is the essential nature of God, the God of whom we are the images, is a love that is replenished right on the spot, in a continuous, reciprocal process of giving and receiving. God's nature teaches us that our refilling can happen during the process of expenditure and can be provided by the one to whom we are giving, by the neighbor we are called to love, by the sufferer we are called to heal.

I mentioned the story of the good Samaritan as a biblical example of the uncalculating liberality of love. The parable is also frequently employed in theological discussions of biomedical ethics to make points about the obligatory—and unilateral—beneficence of the physician, who is pictured in the role of the Samaritan, the one who binds the wounds of the injured man.

In contrast, I shall focus on what I think is the most important—although perhaps the least discussed—teaching point of the parable. What interests me about the story of the good Samaritan is the shifting identity of the neighbor. You remember the setting: Jesus has just agreed with the lawyer that the sum of the law is that we shall love God with all our being and love our neighbors as ourselves. The lawyer then asks the question that triggers the story: "Who is my neighbor?" Jesus tells the story and then asks the lawyer which of the three men described proved to be neighbor to the injured man. The lawyer's answer is the obvious one: the Samaritan, "the one who showed mercy." Jesus responds by telling him to go and do likewise.

With perfectly good warrant, given that injunction, we usually place ourselves in the role of the Samaritan. We are good Samaritans and our neighbors are persons lying injured by the side of the road who require our love and our unstinting aid. However, Jesus' literal answer to the question the lawyer posed requires that we be not the Samaritan, but the injured one. The answer Jesus gives to the question—"Who is my neighbor? Who is this person I am required to love even as I love myself?"—is that my neighbor is the Samaritan, my neighbor is the one who shows me mercy. I am not the Samaritan; I am the one who needs the Samaritan. It is the Samaritan whom I am called upon to love when I am told to love my neighbor.

This is not a pleasant picture. How can I be the helpless, damaged person lying by the side of the road? I am the doctor, I am the minister, I am the healer. I bind up wounds; I do not have them, at least not any wounds that I shall allow to be tended by any Samaritan who comes down the road and happens to find me. Perhaps I do have wounds, but I shall not consider the possibility that they might be soothed by any patient, any parishioner, any needy person who comes by my office, or stumbles into the emergency room, or shows up on the list of people who need visiting. However, when Jesus answers the question, "Who is my neighbor?" he says, in effect, "Picture yourself lying half dead and helpless on the side of the road. Your neighbor—the one you are called to love—is the one who finds you there and tends to you."

Jesus also says, "Go and love your neighbor just as the Samaritan loved the one he found by the side of the road." This is the fascinatingly ambiguous beauty of the parable of the good Samaritan. We can read it both ways. I believe we must read it both ways to understand it: to see that there are two neighbors, two lovers, two inseparably linked facets of the one command to love my neighbor. One is that I must be the Samaritan; I must give; I must show mercy and generous loving care to the neighbors God presents to me. The other is that I must be the injured one; I must receive; I must recognize as my neighbor the one who finds me in my wounded state, and I must love, as much as I love myself, the one who shows mercy to me. My role is always double. If I am to love as God loves, I must be both giver and receiver—and so must my neighbor.

This is not the usual argument that sometimes I am a healer and at other times I am in need of, and must accept, healing. It is, rather, that the healer is always also injured and that the patient is always also one who can heal. I am called to heal and I am in need of healing; the suffering person to whom I minister is the one sent to minister to me.

Several years ago, a fifteen-year-old boy was admitted to the hospital as my patient. He had seemed to be in good health until, suddenly and without warning, he stopped breathing. He was resuscitated and was being supported on a ventilator when he entered the intensive care unit. Our studies quickly showed that the reason for his sudden arrest was a large tumor pressing on his trachea. After several days, our examinations also showed that, although he could now breathe on his own, the damage his brain had suffered from the arrest was severe and irremediable. His tumor could be eradicated with radiation and surgery, but he was likely to remain in a condition just this side of a persistent vegetative state.

Before transferring his care to the oncologist, I had a final talk with his mother to be sure she understood the situation: the cancer treatment would save his life but his brain would probably never recover. I spoke to her with what I thought to be a degree of solemnity and sadness appropriate to the tragic nature of her son's affliction. When I finished, I noticed that she was smiling broadly. She said, "That's all right, honey. I know God's going to raise him up a new body!" Who played the role of Samaritan in this parable? This woman, for whom I fancied myself a sensitive and caring minister, found me in the ditch of hopelessness and brought me back up to her level of wholeness and trust.

This is also not the argument that we may be entertaining angels unaware, that we need to be open to healing from those we serve because one of them may have something important to give us. It is, rather, the argument that we are always entertaining angels unaware. God and God's love, the love that can replace drop-for-drop all the love and mercy we expend, come to us through the mediation of each person God presents us with as an object of our love and service. It works that way because our nature, like God's nature, is relational. Our relations with all our neighbors reflect the relation within the Trinity, defined by constant, mutual giving and receiving. To close ourselves off from that relation, to identify ourselves as healers or ministers only, is, then, to renounce love.

I assume that most of us have little trouble recognizing ourselves as wounded healers, perhaps even acknowledging the importance of our wounded states to the work of healing. It is harder for us to grasp the corollary: that our patients—the ones who suffer, the ones we insist upon serving—are the Samaritan neighbors sent to us to bind our wounds. It is difficult consistently to look upon the sufferers within our community of healing as healers in their own right, as givers as well as receivers in this ongoing dance of mutual neighbor-love, participants in the sort of reciprocity I am speaking of in this chapter.

However, if we are truly to respect, truly to love the suffering ones we serve, we cannot deny them the opportunity to be persons in the fullest sense, the opportunity to enter into relation with us. We must not take away from them their chance, despite their suffering, to remain fully human by being persons who can still give even while they are most in need of receiving. Moreover, if we cannot see them as givers, we cannot understand ourselves as receivers; we too, then, shall not be participating in the dance that defines the universe of God's love.

To make the metaphors of dance and reciprocity less abstract, let us consider what it is that we receive from these neighbors we love, from the patients we doctor, from the suffering ones to whom we try to bring comfort and blessing. How do they show mercy to us?

First, they do so by providing us with the opportunity to love and to serve. They present us with the arena we need for acting out God's command. Richard McCormick has called health care an apostolate, a privileged context in which to encounter another person and, therefore, in which to encounter Christ.[2] This is true not only because we are tending to suffering persons. More important, as an essential part of that care, we are allowed to receive the profoundly significant communication of their selves, their deepest and most feared secrets, the parts of themselves they guard most closely. The ones we serve offer us the unparalleled gift of entry into the hidden life of another human being, where we can hear most clearly the call of God, manifested—as it almost always is—in the person and in the needs of our neighbor. It is the call that bids us to enter, to remain, to understand, to know whom we serve and to know what form that service must take.

When I speak of what patients give us by allowing us "inside," I am reminded of a gripping image of that gracious gift that was depicted in an episode of the television series M*A*S*H. Father Mulcahy, the chaplain, was being interviewed by a journalist. When the camera closed in on him, his face was full of wonder as, with tears in his voice, he recalled seeing the army surgeons, in an unheated operating room in a freezing Korean winter, warming their hands in the steam that rose from the open bellies of their anesthetized patients, warming their hands so they could do their work of healing. The gifts our patients give us are as intimate, as profound, sometimes as unconscious, almost always as mutually beneficial, as the symbolic warmth given and received in that story.

Second, if we listen to them, our patients teach us the natures of their illnesses and the meanings of their sufferings. They teach us our craft and our vocation. They suffer for us as we learn on them, as we literally practice our always imperfect skills. I am sure that not only those of us who are medical professionals, but all of us who minister in any way to the suffering, know, with a certainty that we may or may not wish to acknowledge, that most of what we know about our jobs we have learned from those we have served. The damaged, ailing, sometimes difficult, sometimes endearing persons whom we call patients have all in some fashion taught us how what we learn from books is manifested in the real people God calls our neighbors. To whatever extent we are healers, it is because our patients have made us so.

Third, in shaping us as ministers, those whom we serve

also shape our lives. They form an integral part of who we are; they take a major role in forming our stories as they supply and populate the chapters that follow one another as the narratives of our lives unfold.

There is a popular epigram, generally attributed to John Lennon, that claims that "life is what happens to you while you're busy making other plans." In a similar vein, the Christian apologist C. S. Lewis asserts that what we call interruptions are precisely our real lives, the lives God sends us daily. In the ministry of medicine, the "interruptions" are the people who come to us in need of our service. They, like the people who comprise our families and our circles of friends, are what—or who—happen to us. Our relations and interactions with them form the sum and substance of our lives, giving content and form and meaning to our life stories.

Therefore, it is inevitable and necessary that those whom we serve also give us our wounds. They inflict upon us the vulnerabilities that make possible our service in love's name. They make us fully human, fully one with them. As Robert Coles has explained in his introduction to William Carlos Williams's *Doctor Stories*, they inflict upon us the wounds of presumptuousness and self-importance that seem so inescapable, so incurable for us who are given such daunting power to wield at will.[3] At the same time, they inflict upon us wounds of failure and inadequacy, of ignorance and moral frailty, that make possible the humility that alone can counteract that pride and presumptuousness and keep us faithful to our task.[4]

In forming our stories and in giving us our very human wounds, those who accept our ministrations also shape our characters by their vulnerability. We can be better people because their fragility compels us to be good and gentle and prudent. We can be brave because they are brave, brave sometimes beyond all telling; the courage some show in the face of inexpressible pain and inexorable death can make our own fears seem almost docile by comparison. Insofar as we are just, it is because they need advocates. Insofar as we are trustworthy, it is because they trust us.

"Heal the sick, raise the dead, cleanse lepers, cast out demons. Freely you have received, freely give" (Matt. 10:8). This is the music of God's essential dance of love: freely receive, freely give. We whose lives are bound up with the notion of giving must also receive—freely and openly and fearlessly—God's gifts of knowledge and healing offered to us by the very ones whom we are trying to know and to heal. Then, in turn, we may have within us the power to show God's mercy to them.

❀

CHAPTER 3

SCRIPTURE AS STORY
AND MORAL RESOURCE

The belief that God is Trinity teaches us that the essential nature of love, the love we are called to demonstrate, is mutual self-giving and self-receiving. Loving relationships, like the relation that is the essence of God, are to be constant cycles of that giving and receiving. Belief in a trinitarian God also tells us that, as images of such a God, our natures are also essentially relational. Relationships are part of what constitutes our selves; they are not just adornments to our lives but intrinsic parts of who we are. In speaking of medicine as ministry, this understanding of human nature as relational in its essence has three important implications.

First, our theological, trinitarian orientation teaches us that autonomy, defined as a virtually solitary independence in the language of biomedical ethics, is a chimera. We know that the suffering persons we serve are not served in isolation; each patient we see is comprised to some degree of her relations with other people. To ignore those relations is precisely to violate the integrity, the whole-ness, of that patient. Our understanding of the patient's "autonomy" must be a much richer, more densely popu-lated conception than is commonly advanced.

Second, trinitarian theology insists that the minister, too, is made up of his relations to other people. This as-sertion is in contrast to a narrow, "professional" focus on the job at hand and the illusion of some sort of pure sci-entific objectivity in the person of the healer. No physi-cian, no therapist, no pastoral counselor comes to her work free of the ongoing formative influences wrought by spouses and friends, parents and children, patients and clients.

Third, our theological beliefs call us to see that it is precisely the relation between the one who suffers and the one who wishes to heal that is crucial. This is in con-tradistinction to the ever-present temptation to be de-tached, the temptation for both minister and sufferer to view the other merely instrumentally. Both participants in the healing process are and should be formed to some degree by their particular interaction.

All three of these categories of constitutive relation-ships are essential to the identities of the persons involved in any healing encounter. The third category, the rela-tion between minister and sufferer, is the theme of this book. Moreover, I spoke in the previous chapter specifically about the need for the one ministering to recognize that he receives as well as gives within those relationships.

It is important to stress that the therapist's error of seeing the patient only instrumentally—as only a disease to be diagnosed and treated, only another assignment in one's daily work—can also be committed by the patient. We cannot view those we serve only as so many interesting cases. Likewise, we must ask them not to see us only as useful technicians there to provide prescriptions or sacraments or operations or blessings or flowers from the altar. We must show our patients that healing encounters require the participation of whole persons, and that this includes the whole person of the minister, not just her technical expertise.

I alluded briefly in the previous chapter to the second implication derived from understanding human nature as essentially relational: the importance of the minister's relations to other people, the relations constituting the self he brings to those encounters with persons who suffer. This topic will appear, at various times and in various guises, throughout what follows, affirming our need to maintain our own wholeness so that we may be able to carry out our tasks of ministry within the community of healing.

However, I shall now focus primarily on the idea that the patient's relations to other people constitute her self. We never treat or minister to one person in isolation. We are always serving someone whose very self is inextricably bound up with those others who have been his companions, in one way or another, throughout life. In order to know the person whom we serve—as we must if we are to be healers—we must recognize the relations that have contributed to the construction of that person's self. We must glimpse some part of the rich and complex interweavings that have created the tapestry that constitutes her life and defines her self, the tapestry to which our intervention, our ministry, will also contribute. We must know at least some portion of the patient's story.

There are two different paths along which to develop this idea of the importance of recognizing patients' stories, the narratives of their lives. In the following chapter, I insist that any discussion of the nature of a person's suffering is inadequate, even unintelligible, without the context of that person's story. Suffering can never be anything but meaningless if it cannot be understood as part of one's ongoing narrative. In what remains of this chapter, I interlace the subject of patients' stories with our identification as a Christian community and, therefore, as a community formed by the Story, God's story of creation and fall, incarnation and redemption, steadfast love and mercy: the story we find in scripture.

Scripture is not understood as a list of theological tenets and moral commands handed down by God, inci dentally embellished with some interesting tales to enliven them. On the contrary, theological doctrines and moral precepts gleaned from scripture have no meaning and no authority apart from the story in which they are embedded. The Exodus, for example, is not just a quaint setting for the revelation of self-evident and timeless directives codified as the Ten Commandments. Rather, those commandments can be fully understood, and thoughtfully followed, only when they are grasped as dependent upon and an integral part of the whole story of the people of God, a people defined by that exodus from Egypt, as well as by the golden calf they fashioned, by their anticipation and ultimate attainment of the promised land, by their forty-years' wandering in the desert. The essence of scripture is the story it tells, the whole complicated story.

The nature of God as Trinity teaches us that we, as images of God, are essentially relational. Likewise, the nature of scripture as a narrative that reveals God's way with the world and with us suggests that our way in the world is also in its essence a narrative; it, too, is a story.

It has been said that the basic characteristic of any story is that it has a beginning, a *muddle*, and an end. I have already spoken, and shall speak again, about issues surrounding the ends of our stories. However, most of the time our concerns are about the muddle, the complicated working out of our stories from day to day wherein most of our ethical questions arise. It is in the midst of the muddle that we feel most keenly the need for moral guidance. The story that is scripture is where we, as a Christian community, look for that guidance. Therefore, let us explore briefly what it means to turn to scripture as a moral resource.

To do this we must speak not only of the use of scripture but also of its misuse. In the context of Christian ethics, the misuse of scripture has usually taken the form of a distillation of some set of moral rules from the story the Bible presents, rules that are taken out of context and presented as though they were directly and clearly applicable to moral issues of any time and place. Using the Bible in such a way, as what has been called "revealed morality," presents a number of important difficulties.

First, the extraction of moral rules misses the truly formative ethical content of scripture. As Stanley Hauerwas has explained, the problem of concentrating on biblical texts that look ethical—texts like the Ten Commandments and the Sermon on the Mount—is that such a focus results in far too narrow an understanding of the ethics of the Bible.[1] It separates ethics from the religious and narrative contexts, contexts of creation and fall and redemption, that alone can make an ethical life intelligible or, perhaps, possible.

Second, imputing an abstracted timelessness to the historically situated and shaped words of scripture ignores not only the historical nature of scripture itself but also the truth of the resurrection. Christ's revelation of the nature of God and the meaning of love did not stop with the crucifixion, nor even with the writing of the last book in the canon. In the Gospel of John (5:39–40), Jesus says, "You search the scriptures because you think that in them you have eternal life; and it is they that testify on my behalf. Yet you refuse to come to me to have life." The theologian Arthur McGill built on this teaching when he wrote that "the Scriptures function as a servant of their Lord. We are not meant to rest in them but to move through them and beyond them to the One they serve."[2]

The one they serve is Jesus, and he is not a dead epi-grammatist. He is not Cicero or Marcus Aurelius or Alexander Pope. He did not leave us with nothing more than inspirational couplets. Jesus is alive; it is the living Christ who is our present help in moral discernment. We can derive rules and principles from scripture, but we must not deceive ourselves that they alone are intended to de-termine our actions or to encompass our ethics. Rather, biblical rules and principles are intended to inform and to structure the process of moral discernment that we, as a community centered on the living Christ, are required to undertake. Without such discernment, we limit God to action only in ancient Israel and first-century Palestine as though Jesus had never risen from the dead, and as though we had never received the Holy Spirit.

Another problem in using scripture as a moral source becomes apparent when we engage in that process of moral discernment. There are gaps in scripture: not every moral question has a direct answer in the Bible. A prominent example of the lack of specific answers in scripture to many of our current questions is the favorite bioethical parable of the good Samaritan. Consider the questions one could ask that this story cannot answer, at least not without a lot of creative embellishment.[3]

What if the injured man were still under attack when the Samaritan came along? Should the Samaritan intervene at risk to his own life? Would he be allowed to injure or even kill one or more of the robbers in order to save their victim? What if the Samaritan were a very poor man with a large family to support? Would it be right for him to expend so much money on a stranger? What if he were a physician on his way to see another, critically ill patient, and knew that the delay required to care for the injured man could well mean the death of his other patient, the one with whom he already had a covenant?

What if the injured man also had leprosy? Would the Samaritan be morally required to take care of him even at the risk of infecting himself and his family, as the risk was understood in those times? What if the robbers had attacked a whole caravan, there were dozens of injured persons lying by the road, and the Samaritan had wine and oil and money and donkey space enough to treat only one of them? How would he choose which victim to treat first until he could get to the inn and seek further help, which might come too late for the others?

None of these questions, which closely resemble our current puzzles about the distribution of scarce resources and whether physicians are obligated to treat AIDS patients, is answered in the parable. However, despite these gaps, the parable as it stands does teach us something about the way God would have us love each other that is of infinite importance in the process of moral discernment we bring to bear on our contemporary questions.

We shall not always—in fact, we shall rarely—get from our reading of scripture either direct answers or magical formulas that solve all our ethical problems. Rather, what we shall always obtain there is a dawning understanding of who God is, of how God acts with us, and of how we, therefore, are to act with each other. We shall discover there a vision of what it means to love God and to love our neighbors as ourselves. The growth of that embryonic understanding—our maturation as Christians capable of living moral lives—comes from the hard and sometimes contentious process of working and reasoning together, in the presence of the living Christ, to discern our own scripturally informed answers to our present moral dilemmas.

When Karl Barth claimed that ethical reflection is a matter of repeating the good that has been said, he did not mean that one should simply parrot moral slogans from scripture. "The good that has been said" means the whole truth about God's love and mercy, and about our simultaneous identity as beloved and sinful and redeemed. In ethical reflection our task is to speak that whole truth in language that expresses it fully and faithfully, and in a way that responds intelligibly to the situation on which we are reflecting.

We are not the people of the rules, not the people of the moral code, not the people of the Ten Commandments nor even of the Sermon on the Mount. We are the people of the Book, the people of the Story. To be sure, the story includes those commandments, old and new, but the rules are far from being the whole story.

When I started writing this book, I happened at the same time to read *Kate Vaiden*, a novel by Reynolds Price. There is a passage in it that struck me very forcefully. At one point in her tale, the title character thinks, "Strength just comes in one brand—you stand up at sunrise and meet what they send you and keep your hair combed."[4] I thought that this was just about perfect. Then I quoted it to several of my friends. Each thought it sounded interesting, but none found it as startling and revelatory as I had, and some even seemed to misunderstand its meaning.

I finally realized that the passage's importance and the depth of its meaning stood out for me only because I knew the whole story. In telling me Kate Vaiden's story, Reynolds Price had allowed me to know her and, therefore, to know why her thoughts about strength were so profoundly true. Without the whole story, that passage may make some sense, but it does not have the ring of great and unshakable truth that resonated within me when I read it, nor is it even fully comprehensible.

The same thing is true about statements like "Thou shalt not kill," "Judge not that you be not judged," "Seek ye first the realm of God." These statements make some sense standing alone, but without the whole story told in scripture they are neither fully comprehensible nor fully convincing.

This observation can be extended to statements we hear from the suffering ones we wish to serve, statements like: "I get short of breath," "I don't want any more chemotherapy," "The church has turned its back on my values," "We want to try in vitro fertilization," "Do everything you can to save my father's life." These statements seem at first to be clear and unambiguous; they seem to make some sense standing alone. However, without the whole story of which they are a part, they can be neither fully comprehensible nor fully convincing. Hearing the whole story is the subject of the next chapter.

❄

CHAPTER 4

PAYING ATTENTION

Stories and Suffering

In the preceding chapter, I said we should not read the Bible for lists of rules or for direct answers to most of our specific moral questions. Nevertheless, scripture is a unique and inescapable authority for Christian ethics, although not an absolute judge (only God is absolute).[1] Therefore, let us consider what can be found in our reading of scripture.

There is a long tradition in Christian thought, dating back at least to Augustine (in *De doctrina Christiana*, for example), that teaches us that understanding scripture requires that we come to it prepared to be changed by it.[2] From the standpoint of theological ethics, it is for that change, rather than for any rules or answers, that we go to scripture. Christian ethics, as Richard McCormick has written, is not norms and principles but transformation.[3]

> Do not be conformed to this world, but be transformed by the renewing of your mind, so that you may discern what is the will of God—what is good and acceptable and perfect. (Rom. 12:2)

The crux of biblically informed ethics is that the story of

God's love for us is transformative. It has the power to shape us into the sorts of persons who want and are able to discern what is good, and who then can and will act morally. That story also has the power to shape the church into the sort of community that enables and encourages both the transformation and the empowered action of its members.

To what end is this transformation? There is only one encompassing purpose: to love God with all our being and to love our neighbors as ourselves. The scripture that transforms us comes to us as story, and thereby teaches us to see that our lives and the lives of those we love and serve are also stories and not random collections of disconnected episodes. The transforming story is one that both reveals and compels love. The narrative form of scripture and the agape command that is at the heart of the ethics of the Bible are inseparably intertwined. The story makes no sense without its meaning of love; the love it compels has no content without the narrative that shows us what love is and how love acts.

The metaphor of ever-expanding, ever-clearer vision has long been used in Christian thought to describe this process of transformation, the process of moral and spiritual growth toward the mind of Christ. The more our minds are renewed by the transforming power of God, the more clearly we can see: see what loving God and our neighbor means; see the injured person by the side of the road; see the Samaritan who comes with healing for us; see all the pain, all the suffering that perhaps we would rather not see; see both the infinitely precious object and the incalculably high cost of love. To be transformed is to live and love with open eyes.

In her powerful and painful book on suffering, Dorothee Sölle tells us that, just as freedom from pain is nothing but death, so freedom from suffering is only a blindness that fails to perceive suffering.[4] The truth we must bear, as ministers of medicine, is that we must first see the suffering if we are to help relieve it, and that we cannot see it without in some sense experiencing it. To be transformed, to love with open eyes, is to join in the suffering of the world, as Jesus did.

The story of Jesus' suffering is the basis for the belief that it was his very participation in our pain that makes our salvation possible. Likewise, it is our willingness to see, and thereby to partake of, the suffering of those we wish to serve that makes our service effective.

In love's service there is no substitute for seeing, recognizing, hearing (to use another metaphor) those who are suffering. To acknowledge a sufferer in all her anguish is to begin the process of restoring her to full personhood.[5] In Arthur Miller's play *Death of a Salesman*, Willy Loman's wife seems to understand the crucial role of recognition, for she pleads the case of her desperate husband this way:

"He's a human being, and a terrible thing is happening to him. So attention must be paid. He's not to be allowed to fall into his grave like an old dog. Attention, attention must be finally paid to such a person."[6]

Paying attention to those who suffer—hearing their pain, seeing their damaged selves as damaged selves and not just as vehicles for interesting diagnoses—means, more than anything, listening to the stories they have to tell us. In 1985, Richard Baron wrote a thought-provoking essay in the *Annals of Internal Medicine* titled "I Can't Hear You While I'm Listening." He makes the essential point that we need to take human experience as seriously as we do anatomy and pathology.[7] To do this, we must hear what our patients have to tell us about their experiences.

The more than twenty years I have spent being a doctor have taught me two things that constitute, I believe, the heart of medical practice. One is the importance of the physician's silent presence with those whose lives she or he has changed forever by information and intervention, a presence that allows a true sharing of the burdens of knowledge and fear that pass between healer and sufferer. I shall say more about this silent presence in the final chapter when I speak of the importance of being with the patient through the suffering.

The other thing I have learned is how to take a history—or, rather, how to hear a story. I believe that much of what we teach medical students about taking medical histories from their patients is significantly flawed. We teach them, in effect, how not to listen, how not to hear the human experiences that have brought the patients to seek their help. We accomplish this by teaching the student to force the patient's experience into a prefabricated structure that sorts and separates information in ways foreign to the patient's story as it has been lived.

Anyone who teaches clinical medicine will have observed that hospitalized patients in medical centers often love the green third-year medical students assigned to them, and look upon them as their primary doctors during their hospital stay. I am sure there are many reasons for this phenomenon, but one in particular, I am convinced, is that the students have not yet "mastered" history taking as it is taught to them.

Students are given an enormous list of questions to ask and, usually, some method of selecting the appropriate questions for particular complaints. However, they cannot remember all the questions, and they get nervous, playing doctor for the first time. When they go in to take a history, they often end up just listening to the patient's flow of words, hoping that somehow the answers will appear by chance or that something in the monologue will jog from their memory some question to ask. They do not yet know enough to direct the story into the structured lines that they are taught to use. Consequently, their patients feel that they have finally been heard by someone.

If I were now teaching medical students about taking histories from patients, the first thing I would tell them is that all the lists of questions are to be used, but only to flesh out the story. The questions may clarify details, or stimulate further revelations, or recall a rambling storyteller to the main plot, but they are never a substitute for the story itself. There is much to be learned from the way patients tell their own tales of suffering: what they emphasize, the chronology as they have experienced it, the side events that sound unrelated to us but clearly are not to them, what they fear it all means. Only when we hear all of this can we dare to insert our own questions—about whether a certain symptom is also present, or whether the pain has this or that character—so that the answers fit into the patient's story. Otherwise, the answers create simply our own story: a description of a patient whom we have not heard, a human experience we have not touched.

Understanding illness is mostly a matter of getting the description right, and the description involves far more than just a diagnosis. Diagnosis is one of the extraordinary powers given to physicians, the power of naming. I know, however, that more often than not we get the name wrong, or at least dramatically incomplete. We often get the diagnosis right, but diagnostic labels primarily serve as shorthand tags that physicians find useful for encompassing a theory of pathophysiology and related treatment. A diagnosis is not always a helpful or meaningful label for the illness as experienced by the patient. The following examples illustrate this point.

In Flannery O'Connor's letters, she occasionally spoke of the lupus that was her constant companion and that eventually killed her at the age of thirty-nine. However, when she was very anemic, she did not speak of anemia—much less of bone marrow suppression—as her problem; she spoke of fatigue. When, only a month before her death, she referred to her illness, she did not mention circulating immune complexes, or even nephritis and renal failure. She said simply, "The wolf, I'm afraid, is inside tearing up the place."[8] Her experience was not systemic lupus erythematosus. It was, rather, her awareness of the chaotic, destructive, wolflike gnawing inside that she knew was gradually but inexorably disassembling, "tearing up" her self.

John Updike's story "From the Journal of a Leper" is told by a man who suffers from psoriasis. Although we have learned to laugh at the phrase "the heartbreak of psoriasis," how he describes the disease makes it clear that heartbreak may be a truer name for the illness than the term psoriasis, which he calls "a twisty Greek name it pains me to write." Here is his description:

I am silvery, scaly. Puddles of flakes form wherever I rest

my flesh. Each morning, I vacuum my bed. My torture is
skin deep: there is no pain, not even itching; we lepers
live a long time, and are ironically healthy in other re-
spects. Lusty, though we are loathsome to love. Keen-
sighted, though we hate to look upon ourselves. The name
of the disease, spiritually speaking, is Humiliation.[9]

It is important to get diagnoses right: to recognize psoriasis and lupus, cancer and schizophrenia, AIDS and alcoholism. However, it is no less important to get the name
of the illness right. It is no less important to recognize
that for the sufferer the name of the disease, spiritually
speaking, is humiliation or fear or malaise or endless pain
or loneliness or despair or the end of a career or the end of
a life. It is no less important to recognize that this is a
human being to whom a terrible thing is happening and,
whatever other name this terrible thing bears, its name is
tragedy. There is nothing harder or less sentimental than
Christian realism. Christian realism knows how to call a
tragedy a tragedy, and not some other "twisty Greek name."

Tragedies come in all shapes and sizes, minor and major, but they all have three things in common: they are
sad stories; they have flawed heroes; and they represent
conflicts of good intentions or, more often, gatherings of
evil possibilities.[10]

I have said enough about the importance of stories, and
of recognizing our patients' lives and histories as stories; I

shall not belabor the definition of tragedy as a story. However, I want to emphasize the adjective "sad." Being Christian does not spare us from the sorrow evoked by all that our open eyes see. On the contrary, the concentrated gaze of Christian realism allows us to experience true Christian sorrow[11] with and for those who suffer. This sorrow is not the sentimental, effortless tears we shed for distant starving children on the evening news. It is rather a deep, aching, compelling sorrow that breaks our hearts even while it motivates and empowers our resolve to understand and to love. It is a sorrow that binds us to those we serve as surely as Jesus' tears bound him to Lazarus, Martha, and Mary.

Our sorrow is for the flawed heroes of the sad story, the ones who suffer the action of the tale. "Flawed," in this context, has at least two meanings. Medically, it implies the defect of disease: the disintegration or unwholeness caused by the attack on self-identity that illness inflicts. In a Christian sense, it also implies the imperfection of sinfulness we all bear: sick and well alike, we are all flawed heroes in our own stories.

The word "hero" is at least as interesting. It seems somewhat out of place in the midst of discussion of sad stories and tragic suffering. However, I suggest that identifying sufferers as the heroes within their own stories is a healing move,[12] similar to the healing power evoked by recognition of the complex stories of our patients' lives.

A sometimes difficult corollary of seeing the patient as hero is that the physician is *not* the hero; this adjustment of perspective is probably salutary. We often hear and speak of the heroism of modern medicine, with the term invariably referring to "heroic" actions by members of the medical professions—the desperate fight to save a life with resuscitation techniques, the gallant flight of a transplant team to retrieve a life-saving organ, the dedicated twenty-four-hour efforts of intensive care nurses and doctors. All these people seem heroic; they certainly may be of critical importance to their patients. But they are not the true heroes in these stories.

To do one's job well and thoroughly is an excellent accomplishment, but it is not heroic. To bear the suffering that disease and its remedies bring can be heroic. As William May puts it, "the heavy burden of heroism in medicine falls not on the physician but on the patient and the patient's family."[13] The label of hero belongs only to those who bear the burden of the heroism.

Recognizing the patient as hero should make us think twice about imposing the burden of our own heroics on one who might not choose that particular form of courage. More important, it should add considerably to the reempowering of a person otherwise trapped in the impotence of illness. Such reempowering requires the patient's reintegration, the restoration of his wholeness. It begins with our enabling the patient to regain her voice by our paying attention to her and her story. The process continues with our unwavering recognition of who the hero truly is in this tragedy.

The perception of the true owner and protagonist of the story evokes a much richer sense of patient autonomy than most discussions of medical ethics allow. With our transformed, open eyes we can see the one who suffers as a person in all his wholeness—a person with self-creating relationships and with an intact and meaningful life story into which the present suffering can be incorporated and, therefore, comprehended.

Beyond any minimalist notion of respecting a patient's right to determine his or her own fate, we can now see this burdened hero as the only one who knows all the threads of the story well enough to weave them into the next panel of the tapestry. That panel's colors and textures and design can be congruent with all that has gone before only if the hero who lives within the tapestry, and those who have been allowed to share it, can direct the weaving. Somewhat less metaphorically, it has been said of the patient's autonomy that "the freedom we must honor is not the arbitrary freedom to will one thing one moment and another the next, but the freedom to establish an identity and to maintain integrity."[14]

I speak of "empowering" the patient, but this may have become too glib a catchword. It requires clarification if it is to fit into a specifically Christian ethical proposition. The power I speak of is the gleaming, grueling power that streams through these words of Paul to the Christians at Rome:

> We also boast in our sufferings, knowing that suffering produces endurance, and endurance produces character, and character produces hope, and hope does not disappoint us, because God's love has been poured into our hearts through the Holy Spirit that has been given to us. (Rom. 5:3–5)

"We also boast in our sufferings." This is no frivolous notion of enjoyment, no masochistic reveling in pain. There is too much in scripture and theology to warn us against choosing suffering for its own sake. The solemn "joy" of suffering is only in knowing where it can lead: to endurance, to character, to hope, to the love of God.

"Suffering produces endurance." In the rolling Latin of the Vulgate, this statement is *tribulatio patientiam operatur*, which can also be translated "tribulation produces patience." To be a patient is to be one who is patient, one who endures. To be a patient is to be one who suffers not only in the sense of feeling pain but also in the sense of allowing the pain, of acknowledging and incorporating it as a true thing that is actually happening and that must be dealt with as such. The power of acknowledgment and incorporation—the power to exercise the freedom to establish an identity and to maintain integrity—is the power available to and essential for the suffering ones we wish to serve. It is the power that our recognition of their suffering can evoke and enhance.

It should be clear, then, that in speaking of patience, of endurance, I am not talking about a "stiff upper lip." I am not talking about a foolish, isolating, and fundamentally impotent refusal to admit the presence of pain and to seek its elimination. The stolid, stoical "patience on a monument" that denies its need for healing is not the Christian virtue of patience.

The first known moral essay in Christian history, written around the year 200 C.E. by Tertullian, was entitled *De patientia*, "On Patience." Tertullian makes the pivotal point that the Stoic ideal of patience is designed to result in resignation. In contrast, Christian endurance produces hope. The difference is crucial.

The Christian virtue of patience is the power that looks suffering square in the face, sees it for what it is, and then decides what is to be done about it. It is in this process of clear vision, open acknowledgment, and careful decision that endurance produces character, the sort of character that is full of the hope that neither suffering nor anything else in all creation will ever be able to separate us from the love of God (Rom. 9:35, 39).

CHAPTER 5

❀

WRITING THE NEXT CHAPTER

We who minister to the ill in the name of the faithful community are transformed by the Word of God to be persons who can see. We can now perceive the tragedy that befalls "the patient one" as a sad story centered around a flawed hero. Our perception helps empower in the sufferer a hopeful and virtuous endurance so that she or he also may look upon the tragedy with open eyes and work with us to discern what is to be done, what is, in Paul's words, "good and acceptable and perfect."

It sounds as though we may finally have arrived at the point where we shall have to talk about more traditional medical ethics—about problem solving, about what is to be done. Maybe.

William May, in *The Patient's Ordeal*, makes a distinction, which he attributes to T. S. Eliot, between two sorts of problems. One type of problem raises the question "What are we going to do about it?"; the other asks, "How are we going to behave toward it?" May proposes that many, if not most, of the problems we seek to solve in responding to the suffering of our neighbors are those of the latter sort.[1] For example, if I am coping with the news of a disease likely to be fatal to me, there are things I must do: I must make decisions about therapy, get my affairs in order, and the like. However, these sorts of decisions surely take a back seat to, and in fact depend on, my response to the second question about how I shall behave toward this news. I must first ponder how I choose to conduct the rest of my life in the light of the new, self-shattering information. I must consider how to complete my life in a way that is congruent with who I am and congruent with the way I have lived my life thus far.

The metaphor that leads us to seek "solutions" to our problems may reveal more than we have realized about the intricate process of problem solving. In their book about the largely unnoticed prevalence of metaphorical language in our everyday speech, Lakoff and Johnson tell the story of a young man who was learning to speak English. When he encountered the phrase "the solution of a problem," he adopted with enthusiasm the chemical metaphor that no longer stands out for native speakers familiar with it.[2] His explanation of the image is worth considering as an alternative to the usual notion that to solve a problem is to eliminate it.

When the young man heard "the solution of a problem," he pictured a huge vat of solvent in which problems

76

of various types are suspended. In order to get any particular problem into solution, it is necessary to alter the chemical nature of the solvent. The problem will then become dissolved and seem to disappear. However, if the solvent is altered again, perhaps to handle another problem, the first problem may precipitate; it may come out of solution and, once again, cloud its fluid environment.

Reclaiming the chemical basis of the metaphor of problem solving reminds us that the solution of a problem may at times depend not on its removal but on a change in its environment. "Solutions" may require alterations in the other aspects of one's life that now have to adjust to this new problem in order to fit it in, and thus solve it by assimilating it. It is also worth remembering that later adaptations to newer dilemmas may make old problems reappear, an experience likely to be familiar to most of us.

Some problems, like strep throat or a broken arm, can be eliminated sooner or later. In contrast, many others, like chronic arthritis, alcoholism, cancer, grief—indeed, virtually all the afflictions that entail the kinds of suffering that call for virtuous and hopeful endurance—can find their "solutions" only by being acknowledged and incorporated into the embracing whole of a lifetime's narrative. "Incorporate" is the Latin-based equivalent of the Anglo-Saxon word "embody." What some problems need is embodiment: they need to be given bodies that allow them to fit into the story, forms that are compatible with the story. The rich nuances of the forgotten metaphor embedded in the notion of problem solving can, therefore, lead us toward the adoption of a different metaphor to explain our task. I suggest that we can offer more to those we serve by consciously adopting the metaphor of *story*, so that we can see the process of healing as a process not of solving problems, but of giving narrative form to the events. It is the process of "writing the next chapter."

The stories of all our lives have always been under joint authorship. I may rightly consider myself to be the chief author of my own tale (although, at times, "editor" seems to be the better word, because my life typically happens to me while I am making other plans, and much of my task seems to be to correct the spelling and the punctuation). However, I am well aware that there has been no time when I have been the sole contributor to this work. Parents and siblings, school friends and teachers, children and colleagues, all the people we love and those to whom we commit ourselves—all these people participate in varying degrees in writing the chapters of our life stories. In addition, when a time of medical crisis arrives, the members of the healing community—the pastor and the physician, the comforter and the therapist—will also be part of the composition that solves the problem by continuing the narrative. Together with the family and friends who are old hands at this particular manuscript, they will help the flawed hero embody this newest sad episode within the story of his or her life.

There are several criteria for the writing of that next chapter. First, it has to be part of the hero's story and no one else's. It is undeniably true that our contributions to the stories of those we serve are themselves important parts of our own narratives. However, it is essential that we remember whose crises we are involved in and that we ensure that the paragraphs we add are crafted to fit those persons' tales and not our own.

Second, the next chapter has to make sense. It has to fit the story as it has unfolded to that point. There is no sense in trying to tack the last chapter of *Anna Karenina* onto the first half of *Gone with the Wind*. Scarlett would never have thrown herself in front of a train, even if there had been any railroad tracks left in Georgia, and there is no point in considering such an incongruous outcome.

The meaning of the next chapter must include and somehow continue the themes that have defined the hero's life. This requirement may entail a strenuous examination of previous parts of the story in order for the significance of past activities to be understood, so that the content can be continued even if the activities themselves cannot, because of changes wrought by illness or injury. The process of ensuring continuity may call for an expansion or an altered comprehension of the meanings that animate the story, but such rethinking characterizes healing and growth in their most basic forms.

The work of finding new interpretations and new expressions for the essential meanings of one's life satisfies the third criterion of a good chapter: the new chapter should be able to lead the story on to the other chapters that are to follow. It must be not only continuous with what has gone before but also generative of what is to come: the re-formed, reintegrated life of a whole person.

Sometimes, when the next chapter is actually the final chapter in the story, it leads to the continuation of important threads of the hero's tale in the lives of those who have shared the story. Sometimes the succeeding chapters can be read only in the lives of those left behind to remember and to sustain the meaning of that memory.

The next chapter in the hero's story may be the last chapter, or it may be a chapter so shattering that finding strands of continuous meaning and creative hope seems scarcely possible. To acknowledge this is to recognize once again that the part of the story we are concerned with is indeed a tragedy. Beyond all poetic talk of the tragedy as a sad story about a flawed hero, the fact remains that tragedy is dark confusion and chaos swirling around a conflict of good intentions and, most painfully, a gathering of evil possibilities.

The conflict that characterizes tragedy is perhaps most evident in situations that ask for impossible decisions, situations that seem to need ethics consults. A good example is the case of Debbie, mentioned in the Introduction, in which the good of preserving life comes into uncompromising conflict with the good of relieving suffering, and the evil of failing to respond to pain confronts head-on the evil of ending a life. However, the multiple evils and conflicting goods that create and intensify suffering appear long before that final decision point is reached. It is characteristic of the tragedy of human suffering that it is always a compound insult; the attack is always on more than one front.

Many authors have correctly described illness as an assault on the identity of the patient, or have explained it in terms of damage to the person's wholeness. Others have spoken of a fundamental internal division, a violent separation of the parts of the self that were created to live an integrated life. William May's way of putting it—which I find particularly applicable to an understanding of the communal nature of healing—is that our human identity is best understood in three dimensions: that of the body, our physical presence in the world; that of the community, our relations with each other; and that of the ultimate, our perception of transcendent reality, our connection to God.[3]

With this compound notion of identity, illness can be understood as a simultaneous assault at all three levels, physical, communal, and religious. One conclusion to be drawn from such a perspective is that, to be fully restorative, healing must attend to all three levels. Such an approach affirms the point made in the Introduction that healing involves all segments of the healing community—medical, lay, and clerical. Medicine is a ministry in which doctors are not the only ordinands.

I shall analyze briefly each of these dimensions of healing, and the response to each by the part of the community most closely related to it. However, I wish to make it clear from the start that such a pairing off of the three levels of suffering and the three categories of healers, while it may create neat rhetorical parallels, belies the actual interplay of real patients and real ministers. There is and there should be considerable overlap among these three areas; I do not want my assignment of apparently separate tasks to obscure the complexity of our interactions with those we serve.

Having made this disclaimer, I can say that the physical dimension of illness, which involves a disruption of the patient's unique embodied state in some fashion, is preeminently the domain of the medical professional. It is the obligation of the physician, nurse, or therapist to witness materially to the will of the community to relieve suffering and to reestablish the patient's physical participation in the world of sense, activity, and communication.

Specifically, much can be said about the primacy of the physician's obligation to relieve suffering: to do everything possible to alleviate the illness, to remove the impediment to health, to attend to the patient's physical well-being. One can find innumerable warrants for the doctor's task in scripture, especially in the healing work of Jesus. Although Jesus asked some interesting questions of his patients, he never suggested to them that they would be better off just bearing their pain. Jesus' consistent willingness to relieve physical suffering adds a necessary qualifier and counterbalance to any discussion of the glorious endurance that suffering can produce.

The sort of suffering of which Paul speaks in Romans, the "tribulation that produces patience," must satisfy at least two criteria in order to be productive of the endurance that strengthens character and engenders hope. First, the suffering must be unavoidable. This ineluctability can mean either that the suffering cannot be eliminated—the pain is intractable, the loss irretrievable, the prognosis undeniable—or that what is required for its elimination is unacceptable—a loss of consciousness, say, or a renunciation of deeply held principles.

Second, it must be possible for the suffering in question to produce those goods of endurance and character and hope. There is no point in talking about character building when the torture is so intense and shattering that there may be virtually no self left to be strengthened or to comprehend the idea of hope. Moreover, there is no point in talking about the productivity of suffering when the one who suffers has no discernible capacity to learn from the experience—a person in irreversible coma, for example, or perhaps a newborn infant. As William May writes, "suffering does not always ennoble."[4] It can crush rather than strengthen its bearer.

Therefore, while we recognize and understand the creative potential in suffering, we also know that we are not asked to bear unnecessary suffering. We know that there is some pain that cannot lead to more abundant life. Our Christian hope is built partly upon the assurance that God does not test us beyond our power to endure, but always provides means of escape (1 Cor. 10:13). Such avenues of escape are often under our control. We may not test God's children more rigorously than God would by blocking access to the escape routes God provides.

The suffering that a serious illness inflicts results not only from the assault on the person's physical well-being and sense of embodiment,[5] but also from the threat to that person's relations with those who comprise his or her community. For example, the physician may finally be able to relieve the devastating physical pain of a severe burn, but the psychic pain of permanent disfigurement and its inevitable alteration of relationships does not respond to analgesics. The damage done to a person's self-identification as part of a community can be healed only by the ministrations of that community.

Just as it is the doctor's task to witness to the will to relieve physical suffering and restore the patient's damaged embodiment, so it is the task of the community to witness to the will to sustain relationship with the injured one. In so doing, the community confirms the patient's continued identity as a whole and treasured member. By our refusal to allow suffering to separate the patient from us, we repeat the truth that nothing can separate us from the love of God. We also proclaim an essential fact about human existence, theologically understood: none of the negative aspects of life—sickness and crime and grief and meanness and pain—is absolute in this world. Their elimination is not required for us to be able to live a fully human existence.[6] What is required for a truly human life is not the absence of pain but the presence of others, the maintenance of living bonds with other human beings. It is these relations that are threatened during any self-assaulting illness. As part of their healing, those who suffer require from us assurance that our relationships with them endure.

Sickness is isolating; one of the pains that any serious

illness inflicts is the pain of loneliness. The loneliness cannot be completely overcome, because illness is, ultimately, an intensely personal experience. However, the loneliness that accompanies suffering, though it may still be present, can be stripped of much of its ability to destroy if it is transformed into a sign of the patient's unique and central position within a community that focuses its healing love on him or her.

Flannery O'Connor wrote, "I have never been anywhere but sick. In a sense sickness is a place, more instructive than a long trip to Europe, and it's always a place where there's no company, where nobody can follow."[7] She would probably be quick to acknowledge that she wrote this in a letter to a close friend whose weekly correspondence and frequent visits were part of a network of relationships that kept O'Connor unshakable in her identity and capable of stunningly creative work through all her years of living in that lonely place called sickness. She would also be quick to remind us—and it is important that we not forget—that, despite that supportive network, she could still write this kind of statement and know it to be true.

The third dimension of illness is its assault on one's relation to God. This is the level of suffering to which ordained clergy especially are called to respond. Serious illness shatters our understanding of the way the world works by bringing into question God's power to protect us and even God's love for us.

I considered briefly the possibility of devoting part of this book to questions of theodicy, to the problem we have in reconciling a belief in both God's goodness and God's omnipotence with the obvious presence of evil and suffering in the world. I have chosen, however, not to linger on theodicy, not only because there has already been much written on the subject, most of which focuses appropriately on our misunderstanding of power as an attribute of God, but also because I do not think that it is a particularly helpful emphasis for those who wish to minister to the suffering. None of us wants to be in the role of Job's comforters; we want to be real comforters, real healers. That task requires attention not to the fine points of theological doctrine but to the reality of the patient's experience of pain and to our certainty of God's love.

The theological witness needed to reestablish and reaffirm the patient's relationship to God is the witness of the cross and its double message that evil is real and God is good. It is a message that both validates the reality of the suffering and denies that the pain is absolute. Suffering is real (we cannot accept the stance of Christian Science); suffering may not always be explainable (we are not God, but creatures bound in time); but suffering is not the ultimate reality (we are not lost out here in the stars). And nothing can separate us from the love of God.

Suffering produces hope, "because God's love has been poured into our hearts through the Holy Spirit that has been given to us" (Rom. 5:5). It is, finally, that truth—the truth of God's love in our hearts—that we bring to those who suffer when we treat their bodies, when we sustain our relationships with them, when we assure them that the pain working at them is being vanquished by the love working for them. From these overlapping responses to the several dimensions of illness we can enable in those we serve and in ourselves the transformation of vision that we need, not only to see the suffering itself, but also to see the meaning in the pain.

It is not that the suffering will necessarily make more sense, but that it can now be given form. It can be incorporated, embodied in that next chapter, a chapter that does make sense, that does have meaning. The composition of a next chapter that continues the story's characteristic themes can disclose new possibilities of meaning capable of empowering an uninterrupted, fully human existence even in the presence of the changes illness has caused, or capable of allowing a hopeful, peaceful death and a meaningful next chapter for those left behind.

❀

CHAPTER 6

FOR EXAMPLE
Organ Donation

Thus far I have developed a way of looking at medicine as a ministry that relies on the insights and imperatives of theology and theological ethics, in contrast to the medical model of physician-centered care and to traditional medical ethics. I have proposed that a patient may be better served by an approach that is focused not on problem solving but on the continuation of the narrative of the patient's life, on "writing the next chapter." In this chapter, I clarify both the approaches to medical issues taken by theological ethics, and the way in which a narrative understanding of people's lives plays out in actual decision making. This is a discussion of theological warrants for and decisions about organ donation. It is specifically oriented toward those persons—clergy, laypersons, and medical professionals—whose task it is to counsel individuals considering donation and families debating the decision to allow organs to be taken from loved ones who have died.

Ethics provides many ways to approach the donation

of body tissues and organs. One can analyze issues of justice in the distribution of such a scarce resource, or the thorny problems surrounding the potential use of children or persons in the persistent vegetative state as donors. Here, I explore how we, as theologically directed people, are to understand the possibility of giving away parts of our bodies to other people.

Much theological and, especially, homiletical discourse in favor of organ donation begins with John 15:13: "No one has greater love than this, to lay down one's life for one's friends." Unfortunately, use of the "no greater love" text suggests that the discussion is about the ethics of giving up one's life for someone else. That is not what organ donation is about. When we are asked to donate body organs, we are asked while alive to give up certain parts of the body—blood, bone marrow, a single kidney—whose loss should not kill us despite certain risks in the procedures involved. In addition, we are asked to give more vital parts—heart, liver, both kidneys—only after we are dead. The basic question is not whether we are theologically permitted or even asked to die so that others might live with our body parts. The question is: are we theologically permitted or even compelled to donate parts of our bodies both during life and after death?

In order to consider this question, we must find an appropriate conceptual theological category for the process, a category within which we can reason and through which we can call on resources of scripture and tradition to inform our thinking. We need to place the idea of organ donation within a familiar setting, one that will both reduce the strangeness of the notion and enable us to see more clearly what is at stake. I suggest that an appropriate theological category for the discussion of organ and tissue donation is stewardship, specifically stewardship of the body.

Organ donation can be discussed in terms of the call to love our neighbors as ourselves. However, this command is only what compels us to consider the possibility of donation in the first place. The fact that we are supposed to love our neighbors does not tell us whether giving up parts of our bodies is an acceptable way to show that love. It is not neighbor-love, but how we are to use our bodies, that is the basic theological issue at stake; therefore, stewardship is a fitting category for our thinking about this subject.

Being a steward, in its simplest formulation, means being responsible for both the use and the care of something that ultimately belongs to another. Good stewardship of our bodies is an active and responsible balance of the care and the use of the body; it is the nature of that balance that is relevant to the question of organ donation.

The call to stewardship is a call to recognize a basic fact of our existence: all that we are, all that we have, all that we can do is ours—is under our authority—by virtue of God's creation. We are responsible to God for all that God gives into our keeping, all the time. Stewardship is much more than the commitment of some part of our money to the church for a year. Stewardship is the human condition. Within it we are enabled and expected continually to commit everything to God and to the fulfillment of God's call to love.

Good stewardship of our bodies is something to be discussed and pondered long before the arrival of the crisis point, the moment of stunning loss when the question of organ donation may be raised. Persons suffering through a crushing tragedy can be uniquely receptive to what is said to them at that time, but such situations are not usually the best times for trying to teach an entire way of understanding one's embodied life and its relation to God, and how organ donation might fit into that understanding. The two examples that follow illustrate the futility of expecting families to discuss theology, much less embrace an expanded theological concept of stewardship, at a time of crisis.

Several years ago I cared for a teenage boy who had suddenly fallen victim to an overwhelming infectious process. He died within a few days of his admittance to the hospital. I stood with his family as his mother wept over him, and I heard her say to her dead son over and over again what I have heard so many parents say in that situation: "It's God's will; I know God must want to have you with him." I could not agree with the theology implied in that statement, the terrible and hopeless theology of sticky funeral-parlor sentiments. No loving God would treat us in such a way, and there cannot be any lasting consolation in leaning on a God who would. However, with that grieving family, I knew that it was not the time to initiate a theological discussion about the nature of God's will.

There was another family whose two-year-old daughter drowned in her grandparents' swimming pool. When we talked about the possibility of organ donation, their unanimous and immediate response was to refuse permission because they wished her to go to God with her body intact, as it had been created. It was clear to me then, too, that this was not the time to start a theological discussion about the meaning of bodily resurrection.

Long before the crisis point arrives, we must have come to an understanding of our relation to God and our bodies, and to have wrestled with the notion that organ donation can be an act of the stewardship that defines our lives as God's people. We must teach each other all along about stewardship in a way that will help us understand organ donation as part of a life centered upon the good use and the good care of God's gifts to us. Let us begin by considering what good use might mean.

One of the core biblical teachings about stewardship is the parable of the talents (Matt. 25:14–26), in which three men are given one, two, and five coins to use. The one who hid his talent in order to return it unchanged to the giver is castigated in the strongest terms. Those who invested wisely and doubled the amount of their gift are praised: "Well done . . . enter into the joy of your master."

As many commentators on this parable have noted, an important message to be gleaned from the story is that good use of our gifts requires that we increase their value in some sense. That is, if one has been given intelligence, the gift should in some way be made to grow, perhaps by study and training and then by exercise, to produce other things of value, like a scientific invention or a poem or a sermon.

It is possible to misread this parable as a sort of biblical endorsement of capitalism, especially if we still focus on stewardship as related solely to church budgets. We know money is not the point here, however, any more than good agricultural habits are the point in the story of the sower and the seed. Moreover, what follows the parable makes it quite clear that the sort of stewardship we are called to live is a broad sort indeed. The story that comes next in Matthew's string of descriptions of the realm of God is the story of the sheep and the goats (Matt. 25:31–46).

In the parable of the talents, it is the person who doubles

94

the master's gift of money who is welcomed into the joy of the kingdom. In the following story, that same joyful reception is accorded to those who have fed the hungry, who have sheltered the stranger, who have clothed the naked and visited those who are sick or in prison. "Come, you that are blessed by my Father, inherit the kingdom prepared for you from the foundation of the world." This story can help interpret what our "talents" are and what it means to increase their value.

We have been given compassion and intelligence, the ability to teach and to heal, the means to keep ourselves well fed and clothed and sheltered, the opportunity to enter into relation with other people. We may increase the value of these gifts by cultivating them, surely, by study and effort, but also by using them to teach, heal, feed, clothe, shelter, and be present with those who need what we have to give. We enhance the value of our own gifts by attending to our neighbors.

We have also been given a physical body, which, even more than our other gifts, is inseparably identified as "us." Our body is the bearer and expresser of all our gifts. We increase the value of our body by caring for it, surely, by attending to its needs and concerns, but also by using it to honor those we are called to love. It is in the body that we bring food to the hungry, that we visit the sick and the captive. It is through the body that we touch those we wish to heal and speak with those we wish to teach. It is as uniquely embodied persons that we enter into relation with the neighbors God calls us to love. When the opportunity arises, we can sustain those in need in an even more intimate fashion by giving parts of our bodies so that others might be healed.

It is entirely in keeping with the spirit of the parable of the talents and the story of the sheep and goats to extend their joint allegorical meanings to include the sort of stewardship that organ donation entails. "I was hungry and you gave me food." I was bleeding to death and you gave me your blood. My heart was failing and you let me have the strong heart of your child who was brain dead after an auto accident.

A theological, scriptural understanding of stewardship and of our relation to our bodies as stewards unquestionably affirms and encourages donations of parts of our bodies to those who need them so that they may continue to live, or may see again, or may be restored to physical wholeness. God has given us these bodies so that we might live in this world in loving relation with each other. Organ donation is a profoundly important way in which we can do this.

In addition to declaring that organ and tissue donation in itself is a good expression of stewardship, we also have the theological task of dispelling some sentimental and superstitious ideas that often cloud the issue or even act as barriers to good stewardship.

One sentimental notion that needs to be abandoned is the phrase that for many years has permeated talk of organ donation. For too long, organ donation has been described as the "gift of life." Let us be very clear about this. God gives life. No body part of mine or yours, no matter how vital, gives life to anyone else. What donation does is to make possible the continuation of life in one who would otherwise die, or the enhancement of life in one who would otherwise be trapped in the sort of suffering, such as that associated with chronic dialysis, blindness, or disfigurement, that threatens to diminish life.

Organ donation is an excellent gift. It does not need to be overdramatized into a godlike act of creation in order to make it seem good. It is an act of love and faith that should be as normal a part of loving our neighbors as feeding and clothing and visiting them.

We must also clear away superstitious ideas about what is meant by the resurrection of the body. In the earliest years of Christianity, apologists were forced to come to terms with this question because of the incredulous ridicule of pagan critics who found the notion absurd. Those critics correctly pointed out the problems created by persons who died in the desert and were picked apart by vultures, or who died at sea and were nibbled by fishes. What of the believer whose body had been torn to pieces by the lions in the Colosseum? How did the body re-form? How could believers be taken seriously?

The answers to such questions were hammered out with variable degrees of success during the first centuries of this era, but the questions keep recurring. Now, however, the questioners are the believers—not the critics. Like the parents who wanted their drowned daughter to go to God intact, some will say, "How can I let them take the organs from my son when that means he will have to go through eternity with such a damaged body?"

This kind of misunderstanding cannot be challenged in the midst of the shock and grief of death, when organs are being requested. Rather, we must first seek to educate through our teaching of the Christian view of bodily resurrection, based on Paul's statement that we shall be changed and that what is sown corruptible will be raised incorruptible. We believe that we shall indeed be embodied in some fashion throughout eternity, maybe even in a way that is reminiscent of our earthly form. However, there is nothing in scripture or the traditional teachings of the church to suggest that the exact structure that comprises a bodily existence will somehow be translated, molecule for molecule, into eternity.

There is a more important obstacle that stands in the way of the donation of organs, particularly donation from the body of a deceased family member. This obstacle deserves our careful attention and respect.

For many years I cared for a lovely little girl, whom I shall name Anna, who had leukemia. Nothing in Anna's treatment ever came easily; she seemed to have every complication imaginable. Eventually, after years of stubborn fighting, she died late one night after a fierce, brief battle with infection. As I went through all the paper-signing formalities with her parents, I turned toward them to make the usual request for an autopsy. Before I said a word, Anna's father, a pediatrician, raised his hand to stop me. While Anna's mother, a nurse, nodded her agreement, he said, "I know what you're going to ask; I've asked it a hundred times myself. I know all the reasons why I should say yes, but I can't. All I know is that she has suffered enough. There's not going to be anything else done to her body. No autopsy."

I did not argue with him. I did not tell him she could not suffer any more. I did not tell him that it was his suffering he was trying to assuage, not his daughter's. Such statements may have been true, but they were irrelevant. What Anna's father was telling me was that her body was now to be honored and cared for and protected—in a way that he and her mother had not been able to do during all those years of allowing her to be punctured and irradiated and poisoned in the hope of a cure.

In Anna's case, the question was one of autopsy, but the family's response—that she had suffered enough—is heard as often in situations where organs are being requested. In each instance, the proposal is to cut into the body and remove some part of it. In each instance, the claim that the deceased person is capable of further suffering may be a metaphorical way of expressing the family's deeply felt need to protect and honor the physical remains of the person they loved. The body represents, in a way beyond photographs and memories, the lived existence of that person. It can be very difficult to allow that body to be altered. In fact, we often go to great pains to ensure that the dead body makes its final journey looking well cared for and even well dressed.

The claim that one who has died is still capable of suffering may also be a way of saying that the suffering of the one who has died and the suffering of those left behind are connected. There is a sense in which Anna's pain and her parents' suffering are inseparable, perhaps even indistinguishable.

There is nothing simple or irrational about such an understanding of our interconnectedness with those we love. It is not to be dismissed as insignificant, or derided as superstitious, or violated as trivial, even when compared with the critical needs of those awaiting transplants. Our task is to help those we counsel find an appropriate balance between the profoundly good need to honor and protect our bodies and the bodies of those we love from injury and invasion, and the profoundly good need to give our body parts and those of our loved ones to others whose lives may depend upon our gifts. This is the balance of good stewardship, the balance we have to seek between good care and good use of what we are and what we have. In short, we must be sure we do not become so enamored of the undeniable good that organ donation accomplishes that we dishonor both the body and the life of the donor. The goodness of organ donation cannot be assumed always to override the other goodnesses to be sought in our care for the dead.

I have an aunt who has always had definite opinions on what one may and may not do with dead bodies. Once, when I was young enough to think it clever to bait my elders, I challenged her about why it should make a difference, once she is dead, if her body is thrown to the sharks. She, long the faithful tender of the family graves, was horrified at the thought. She could not bear the idea of her body not being preserved intact, inviolate, within her place in the family burial plot.

I use this example to stress the importance of honoring a person's beliefs and wishes after she or he has died. It is not important whether or not the person's convictions on this subject appear entirely rational. What is important is that the person be honored in death as in life. I could not imagine giving permission for organs to be retrieved from my aunt's dead body or even for an autopsy to be performed. Either would be a disavowal of the person she has been and the wishes she has repeatedly expressed.

The part of stewardship that is good care ultimately means putting "good use" in the context of the entire story of the person's and the family's life. To give permission for organ donation from my aunt's body would be to violate the story of her life. Donation under those circumstances could not be considered good use of her body, the body that is an inseparable part of the story that defines her. I might wish it were otherwise; I might wish she lived the sort of life that could be appropriately capped with the gift of a body part after death. However, my primary obligation is to honor her in her death, not to rewrite her life.

Our lives are stories. They are ongoing narratives that flow through time. They are defined by threads of continuous meaning, expressed in our actions and in our connections. We do not live discrete moments in time. We do not experience life as one disconnected event following another. We do not live schematic biographical outlines that jump from birth to school to work to marriage to children to death.

Rather, we live our lives as continuous narratives, as streams of relationship and activity that read like a novel and not like a list. All the characters and all the happenings are interwoven and influence each other. They all have meaning only within the whole story. Time does not stand still, not even at the most dramatic points in our lives. The story goes on and incorporates all those events into its flow. And the point that marks the end of a life is part of that ongoing story.

The decision to be an organ donor should be congruent with the entire narrative of one's life if one is to maintain integrity. However, if such a decision appears incongruent—if it comes, for example, from someone who otherwise seems to be a crabby miser—this does not mean the offering should be rejected. The goodness of the message does not depend on the goodness of the messenger. I doubt that anyone at the Red Cross cares whether or not a blood donation comes from a cheerful giver. My point is, rather, that we who are theologically directed must call each other into lives of stewardship within which the donation of body parts can make sense.

If my life were characterized by generosity and compassion, it would be appropriate for my story to include a decision to donate certain tissues now. It would also make sense for me to want to give organs after death and, therefore, to do now the legal work necessary to ensure that that can happen. Organ donation has to be an integral part of my overall understanding of my life, if I am to preserve my integrity as a whole person with a meaning-ful life—and if I am to enable those who love me to honor my identity and maintain my integrity after my death.

Many times people die without having expressed their beliefs or wishes about organ donation. In such a situation, the decisions made by those who have known the person best should be arrived at within the context of that person's life. As we talk with the grieving family and friends, our task may be to help them replay the story, to find the threads of meaning in it—the passions and creeds and loves that ran through all the years, all the chapters—so that they can then compose a final chapter that fits the rest of the story. I hope that my friends and family, if they were called on to write my concluding chapter, would see that organ donation from my body would be an appropri-ate way to end my story—a final act of deep giving and a final statement of mutual relation that would echo the giving and relationships that had marked my life to that point.

However, there are those whose lives and beliefs make organ donation unthinkable, perhaps because of deep-seated fears of bodily violation that have haunted them throughout their lives, or strongly held beliefs about the resurrection of the body, or a profound aesthetic repug-nance to the idea of sharing body parts. The specific rea-son is immaterial; whether or not we find it comprehensible is not important. When such a person dies, it can only be hoped that the family will have the sense and the courage to honor his or her life by refusing organ donation. Moreover, we must support and respect them in that decision.

Yet there is a way in which we can attempt to counteract the revulsion some feel at the idea of giving organs, to counteract the fear that to allow organ retrieval is to dishonor the body and even to increase the pain of death.

The primary way in which we honor the body of a deceased person is to dispose of it by the meaningful, liturgical process of a funeral service. It is possible to draw analogies between the meanings of a funeral and the meanings of organ donation that demonstrate that donation is as much an act of profound respect for the body as is a funeral remembrance.

The most obvious analogy is that both a funeral and organ donation after death acknowledge that the person's life is at an end. Death is a real and lasting separation. Funerals bring closure and finality to a life, allowing the final statement of that life to be made within the community that sustained it. Organ donation, in similar fashion, seals the person's life with a final, permanent act of mutual relationship. It is an act that, like a funeral service, frames the final proclamation that perhaps we would all like to be the last words we hear: "Well done."

A funeral is more than a forceful reminder that the life

of someone we have cared for is over. It is also an expression of the continuation of that person's life within the ongoing lives of family, friends, and community. It is an expression of the robust interconnectedness of us all. To say farewell in a ritual manner is to acknowledge the importance of that life, to give it both a completion and an extension, to imprint it in the memories and the living histories of those present.

As the older members of my family die, it is at their funerals that I and the other members of my generation recognize and accept the cycle that is moving us from the youngest to the oldest levels of this continuous and interwoven yarn of human existence. At those times, we also recognize and accept the traces we bear of those who have left first. This cousin has our aunt's high forehead, that one our grandfather's skinny neck; another cousin now looks much as her mother did at that age. It seems to be especially at funerals that we stand together and talk quietly of all these things, and see our common memories written on our bodies.

The continuity and interconnectedness of life that funerals acknowledge can be just as clearly manifested in the act of organ donation. Giving the heart or the kidney or the liver of someone you have loved in order to sustain the life of another is, in a profoundly moving way, to continue the memory of that loved person. It is to sustain the presence of that person within the human community in a fashion more vibrant than the placement of a stone in a cemetery or even the establishment of a college scholarship. Perhaps more accurately, it is to be able to say, with equal precision, "My new nephew has my father's eyes, but so does the young woman who was blind until she received the gift of his corneas."

Because funerals are statements of our continuity and connections with each other, they are also expressions of hope for the future: hope for the resurrection of the one we love, and especially a hopeful confidence in the goodness and future of humanity. Of all the awful scenes associated with the Holocaust, I find few more terrible, more bereft of hope, than the photographs of mountains of human bodies piled in the trenches that served as graves. The apparent absence of acknowledgment of those deaths as they occurred—however minimal and halting any ritual would necessarily have been—is such a bleak statement of hopelessness because it insists that life is meaningless, that there is no reason to wish it to continue, that no matter what effort you make, what love you give and receive, what music you sing, life ends in a trash heap.

The ritual of a funeral says just the opposite. It is a celebration of human life, a commemoration of precisely the efforts one has made, the love one has shared, the music of one's life. It is the ultimate statement that it does matter that we have lived here and, therefore, that it does matter crucially that human beings will continue to live here, and work, and love.

The positive and even joyful statement about the goodness and importance of human life that is proclaimed in a funeral service is echoed and amplified in the gift of part of one's body to ensure the continued, healthy existence of another member of humanity. In this sense, the gift of an organ, like a funeral, is an affirmation, in the face of all that is difficult to affirm in this life, in the face of poverty and cruelty and pain and inexorable death, in the face of the suffering and death of the donor. It is an affirmation of the intrinsic goodness of living and of the desire that human life continue.

A funeral and the donation of an organ are forms of witness. They are faithful witnesses to the life of the community, to the endurance of love and life itself beyond the power of death to threaten them. They are witnesses to the integrity and meaning of the entire life of the one who has died. Each contributes its own poetry to the final stanza of that life's story of trust and hope.

CHAPTER 7

❃

RITUALS OF HEALING

Given the importance of reciprocity in the relationship between patient and minister, it is necessary to acknowledge the suffering that afflicts those of us who seek to serve the sick. Thornton Wilder's brief play *The Angel That Troubled the Waters* is an imaginative expansion of the biblical story of the healing pool at Bethesda (John 5:2–9). In Wilder's version, a physician comes to the pool in search of healing for himself. One of the invalids who spend their days there, awaiting the angel's touch that will transform the waters into balm, tells him it is no place for a healer, especially one who is obviously so healthy. The angel then appears, visible only to the physician, and tells him,

> Healing is not for you. . . . Without your wound where would your power be? It is your very remorse that makes your low voice tremble into the hearts of men. The very angels themselves cannot persuade the wretched and blundering children on earth as can one human being broken on the wheels of living. In Love's service only the wounded soldiers can serve. Draw back.[1]

The invalid who rebuffed the physician jumps into the now-troubled water and is healed.

This play is more than a little troublesome. It is a moving and probably valid claim that "in love's service only the wounded soldiers can serve." This notion has been expressed in many different ways by theologians and physicians and poets. But what of the angel's saying to the one who serves the sick that healing is not available for the server?

Even if we are better able to serve because of our frailties, can it be true that there is no healing for us? Are we to be turned away when we seek relief from the pain that our service causes us? What scripture teaches about God's healing, and my own experiences of restoration, tell me otherwise. There is healing for the physician in Wilder's play, but not in the stirred-up waters. The healing that happens in the pool at Bethesda is not for the healer, because the healer's relief is to be found in communion with those who work alongside the healer and in communion with the ones whom together they serve, not in the solitary refreshment of a direct divine touch. The minister's wounds, having been inflicted by the faithful act of being in community, are healed within that faithful community.

In Chapter 2, I referred to the reciprocal, giving-and-receiving nature of Christian existence. As givers who also receive, we know that the tragedies we confront as ministers of healing are also, in some sense, tragic events in our own lives. That is, in the act of ministry, the sufferings we seek to relieve cannot help but cause us to suffer to some degree. Our relations with each other are that closely intertwined; Paul was correct when he said that we are to "bear one another's burdens" (Gal. 6:2).

Like our patients, we are also exhorted to rejoice in our sufferings, in the privilege of sharing the burden. We are to rejoice not only in giving but in receiving the healing love of the community. That love can empower in us, too, the endurance that can produce a character full of hope in the love of God that does not allow suffering to divide us. In Wilder's play, the invalid who has just been healed praises God, prays for the physician's healing, and then invites the physician back out of his solitary pain and into his place within the community. That is where we find our healing: where our work is, where our love acts.

Those who do the work of medicine cannot endure the vocation without the continued healing support of the entire community whose task is the relief of the suffering in its midst. That community is defined not only by its job of healing but also by its primary identification as God's people. Our conscious and ever-renewed rootedness within God's community is finally what allows us to experience and to survive the pain of drawing so close to the suffering persons we serve. As David Barnard has written, "The conviction that we are 'held,' in an ultimate sense, validates every particular embrace, and finally permits every letting go."[2]

In Chapter 5, I made a distinction between two sorts of problems, noting that the suffering that needs the healing touch of the ministering community is usually the type that needs not a finite solution but a certain orientation, a kind of conduct by which to live with the problem fruitfully. This perspective implies that the sort of behavior required of us in approaching suffering may be less a technical operation than a ritual enactment, a moral and aesthetic process of revelation and remembering, accomplished within the community of faithful ones.

The performance of communal rituals of healing identifies the ministry of medicine as liturgy. Vigen Guroian, a theological ethicist of the Eastern Orthodox church, reminds us that the Greek origin of the word *liturgy* "connotes an action through which persons come together to become something corporately which they were not as separate individuals."[3] The ministry of medicine is the liturgy through which healers and sufferers become corporately the community in which healing love can act.

Much of this book describes, in one way or another, rituals that comprise the specific liturgy of medicine. The process of composing jointly the next chapter of the patient's life is perhaps the central ritual around which the healing community gathers. In my own experience, there are two other healing rituals within the practice of medicine that have also served to sustain me in the work of ministry. One is the ritual of taking a history, of letting the story of suffering unfold, as described in Chapter 4. This is a service that happens not just at the beginning of my encounter with a patient, but each day of the illness, as I listen again and, perhaps, become more of a contributor to the story. In this way, the history undergoes its gradual metamorphosis from a story of the past to a description of the present to a speculative projection of the future, and the content of the next chapter takes shape in this ritual of dialogue and communion.

The other sustaining, healing ritual is something I can only call "the ritual of being there." It is the solemn act of being present with the child as she struggles with her new knowledge, with the family after I tell them the shattering news, with the patient as he dies, with the parents as they hold their infant for the last time. It is often difficult to remain fully present at times of such searing pain, but there are at least two reasons that compel me to stay. One is the moral necessity of not only declaring the crisis—by making the diagnosis, pronouncing the death—but seeing it through in all its awful reality. The privilege of accompanying my patients through the risky journeys of illness includes the obligation to walk with them on the grim paths of pain.

I feel compelled to be present also because, during those silent, suffering vigils, I learn what I could never know were I to walk away after doing my technical job. I learn more about the ministry of medicine than I can find in textbooks. There was the twelve-year-old girl whom I had to tell that the disease she had been fighting for the last six weeks was leukemia, and that it was now in remission. After a long period of silence, she responded with the wail, "But that means it can come back!" She taught me in a flash the difference between my perception of a disease in remission and her experience of a devastating illness waiting to return.

There was the mother mourning the death of her son. She was an older woman, a widow. Fifteen-year-old Nick was her youngest child; all her other children were much older, grown and gone. She and Nick lived alone together. He had a huge brain tumor, and he progressed from his first bad headache to being brain dead over a period of less than twenty-four hours—an incomprehensible lightning strike of tragedy. I pronounced him dead and took him off the ventilator. His mother sat in a rocking chair by his bedside in the intensive care unit and wept quietly. I stood at the foot of his bed, saying nothing.

After several minutes, she started mumbling, and then

she began talking louder and more distinctly as her litany of mourning became stronger, matching the rhythm of her rocking. At what seemed to be the peak of her keening, she turned to me and articulated her grief in precise terms. She asked, "Who's going to sit on the porch in the evening with me? Who's going to go to the grocery store with me?" I had no answer but my own tears.

By being there, I learned—in a way that nothing else could have taught me—exactly what that loss meant in that woman's life. I learned the depth of her wound, the lonely dread that would now shadow the composition of her next chapter. I also believe that, by being there, I gave her the human companion she needed for a partner in her groping attempts to give voice to the meaning of her grief, her own very particular loss. Giving suffering its voice is the beginning of healing.

Hearing the story and being present through the suffering are rituals that can sustain and enable medicine as ministry in crucial ways. There are many others of importance, like medical rituals of the laying on of hands in the physical examination, sacramental rituals of anointing and prayer and reconciliation, ministering rituals of visitation and providing for the families of the ill. All of these find their roots and their meanings in the primary ritual of the Christian community: the rite of communion, the eucharist.

All that I have discussed in this book is grounded, affirmed, and empowered in the liturgical act of communion. The service of the eucharist is a teacher and protector against the idolatry that tempts us daily, for it recalls us to the reality in which God is God and everything else is not. In the eucharist we participate in the prototype of the giving-and-receiving reciprocity of love that defines the essence of God. We present ourselves, souls and bodies, as a living sacrifice to God and, at the same time, take in the very life of God that, in Jesus, was broken and poured out for us so that we might be part of the love that God is.

The act of communion confirms, even as it defines, our essential interrelatedness, the truth that our selves are constituted in part by our connections to each other. By participating together in our communion with God, we remember that our relations with each other are mirrors of God's triune nature: we are images of the resonating love that overcomes evil. We know then that it is only our love for each other that can finally overcome our suffering.

It is in the liturgy of the eucharist that scripture and ethics meet.[4] In it, we reenact the story of creation, fall, and redemption, consciously placing ourselves within the long history of salvation, identifying ourselves as the people of God. By doing so, we receive the understanding and the courage we need to act as God's people in the world.

The eucharist is an experience of drawing close to God and finding God drawing close to us, again and again, through all the weeks of our lives—despite what those laboring weeks contain of sin and suffering, of technical success and moral failure, of consuming pain and illusory hope. In that experience we can reclaim our certainty that nothing can separate us from the love of God and the unshakable conviction that we are indeed held in the arms of God and in the arms of God's people. That conviction validates every particular embrace, every individual searing exposure to the real and devastating tragedies that human beings experience. That conviction finally also permits every letting go, every release of incomprehensible suffering into the limitless expanse of God's mercy.

NOTES

❀

INTRODUCTION

1. Stanley Hauerwas, *Suffering Presence* (Notre Dame, Ind.: University of Notre Dame Press, 1986), 78–82.

2. "It's Over, Debbie," *Journal of the American Medical Association* 259 (8 January 1988): 272.

I. GOD IS ONE: THE TEMPTATIONS OF IDOLATRY

1. Alasdair MacIntyre, "Theology, Ethics, and the Ethics of Medicine and Health Care," *Journal of Medicine and Philosophy* 4 (1979): 435.

2. David Barnard, "Religion and Medicine," *Soundings* 68 (1985): 455.

3. Reinhold Niebuhr, *An Interpretation of Christian Ethics* (San Francisco: Harper and Row, 1935), 53.

4. Georges Bernanos, *The Diary of a Country Priest* (New York: Macmillan, 1937; repr., New York: Carroll and Graf, 1983), 11.

5. Flannery O'Connor, "A Good Man Is Hard to Find," in *The Complete Stories* (New York: Farrar, Straus, and Giroux, 1971), 133.

6. Dietrich Bonhoeffer, *Ethics* (New York: Macmillan, 1965), 84–85.

7. Joseph Fletcher, *Situation Ethics: The New Morality* (Philadelphia: Westminster Press, 1966).

8. Flannery O'Connor, *The Habit of Being*, ed. Sally Fitzgerald (New York: Random House, 1980), 90. The meaning of the phrase "Christian realism" is clarified by the context of O'Connor's

statement. In response to critical reviews that labeled one of her stories "brutal," she wrote: "The stories are hard but they are hard because there is nothing harder or less sentimental than Christian realism. I believe that there are many rough beasts now slouching toward Bethlehem to be born and that I have reported the progress of a few of them." Christian realism, in her letter and in this book, in contrast to more political usage, refers to an unflinching view of human beings as deeply flawed creatures who are both burdened by and capable of inflicting suffering, and who nevertheless can be recipients of grace.

9. Karl Barth, *Church Dogmatics* (Edinburgh: T. and T. Clark, 1961), II.2.537.

10. Ibid., III.4.324.

11. Niebuhr, *Interpretation of Christian Ethics*, 131.

2. GOD IS THREE: METAPHORS OF RELATION

1. An exceptionally thoughtful and lucid exposition of the Trinity as relational is given by Elizabeth A. Johnson in *She Who Is: The Mystery of God in Feminist Theological Discourse* (New York: Crossroad, 1994), 191–223.

2. Richard A. McCormick, "Theology and Bioethics: Christian Foundations," in *Theology and Bioethics*, ed. E. Shelp (Dordrecht, Netherlands: D. Riedel Publishing Company, 1985): 108–9.

3. Robert Coles, introduction to *Doctor Stories*, by William Carlos Williams (New York: New Directions, 1984), xiii.

4. William F. May, "The Virtues in a Professional Setting," *Soundings* 67 (1984): 245–66.

3. SCRIPTURE AS STORY AND MORAL RESOURCE

1. Stanley Hauerwas, "The Moral Authority of Scripture: The Politics and Ethics of Remembering," *Moral Theology* No. 4, *The*

Use of Scripture in Moral Theology, eds. Charles E. Curran and Richard A. McCormick (New York: Paulist Press, 1984), 247.

2. Arthur C. McGill, *Suffering: A Test of Theological Method* (Philadelphia: Westminster Press, 1968), 30.

3. James F. Childress, "Love and Justice in Christian Biomedical Ethics," in *Theology and Bioethics*, ed. E. Shelp (Dordrecht, Netherlands: D. Riedel Publishing Company), 225–26.

4. Reynolds Price, *Kate Vaiden* (New York: Ballantine Books, 1986), 108.

4. PAYING ATTENTION: STORIES AND SUFFERING

1. James M. Gustafson, introduction to *The Responsible Self*, by H. Richard Niebuhr (New York: Harper and Row, 1963), 22.

2. Charles M. Wood's *Formation of Christian Understanding* (Valley Forge, Pa.: Trinity Press, 1981) teaches much the same lesson as Augustine.

3. McCormick, "Theology and Bioethics," 102.

4. Dorothee Sölle, *Suffering* (Philadelphia: Fortress Press, 1975), 37–39.

5. Howard Brody, *Stories of Sickness* (New Haven, Ct.: Yale University Press, 1987), 125.

6. Arthur Miller, *Death of a Salesman*, in *The Portable Arthur Miller*, ed. Harold Clurman (New York: Viking Press, 1971), 50.

7. Richard J. Baron, "An Introduction to Medical Phenomenology: I Can't Hear You While I'm Listening," *Annals of Internal Medicine* 103 (1985): 606–11.

8. Flannery O'Connor, *The Habit of Being*, ed. Sally Fitzgerald (New York: Random House, 1980), 591.

9. John Updike, "From the Journal of a Leper," in *Problems and Other Stories* (New York: Alfred A. Knopf, 1979), 181.

10. Hessel Bouma et al., *Christian Faith, Health, and Medical Practice* (Grand Rapids, Mich.: Eerdmans, 1989), 124–32.

11. McGill, *Suffering*, 115–18.

12. Rita Charon, "Doctor-Patient/Reader-Writer: Learning to Find the Text," *Soundings* 72 (1989): 147.

13. William F. May, *The Patient's Ordeal* (Bloomington: Indiana University Press, 1991), 3.

14. Bouma et al., *Christian Faith*, 15.

5. WRITING THE NEXT CHAPTER

1. May, *Patient's Ordeal*, 3–4.

2. George Lakoff and Mark Johnson, *Metaphors We Live By* (Chicago: University of Chicago Press, 1980), 143–44.

3. May, *Patient's Ordeal*, 9–12.

4. Ibid., 50.

5. "Embodiment" here is not intended to signal the varied philosophical and experiential nuances that the term carries in, for example, feminist thought. In the context of this book, embodiment refers simply to the fact of human physicality, especially as it seizes our attention in situations of pain and disease.

6. Ibid., 153.

7. O'Connor, *Habit of Being*, 163.

7. RITUALS OF HEALING

1. Thorton Wilder, *The Angel That Troubled the Waters* (New York: Coward-McCann, Inc., 1928), 148–49.

2. Barnard, "Religion and Medicine," 463.

3. Vigen Guroian, "Seeing Worship as Ethics: An Orthodox Perspective," *Journal of Religious Ethics* 13 (1985): 334.

4. Vigen Guroian, "Bible and Ethics: An Ecclesial and Liturgical Interpretation," *Journal of Religious Ethics* 18 (1990): 129–57.

BIBLIOGRAPHY

❀

Barnard, David. "Religion and Medicine." *Soundings* 68 (1985): 443–65.

Baron, Richard J. "An Introduction to Medical Phenomenology: I Can't Hear You While I'm Listening." *Annals of Internal Medicine* 103 (1985): 606–11.

Barth, Karl. *Church Dogmatics*. Edinburgh: T. and T. Clark, 1961.

Bernanos, Georges. *The Diary of a Country Priest*. New York: Macmillan, 1937; reprint, New York: Carroll and Graf, 1983.

Bonhoeffer, Dietrich. *Ethics*. New York: Macmillan, 1965.

Bouma, Hessel, et al. *Christian Faith, Health, and Medical Practice*. Grand Rapids, Mich.: William B. Eerdmans, 1989.

Brody, Howard. *Stories of Sickness*. New Haven, Ct.: Yale University Press, 1987.

Charon, Rita. "Doctor-Patient/Reader-Writer: Learning to Find the Text." *Soundings* 72 (1989): 137–52.

Childress, James F. "Love and Justice in Christian Biomedical Ethics." In *Theology and Bioethics*, edited by E. Shelp, 225–44. Dordrecht, Netherlands: D. Riedel Publishing Company, 1985.

Coles, Robert. Introduction to *Doctor Stories*, by William Carlos Williams. New York: New Directions, 1984.

Fletcher, Joseph. *Situation Ethics: The New Morality*. Philadelphia: Westminster Press, 1966.

Guroian, Vigen. "Seeing Worship as Ethics: An Orthodox Perspective." *Journal of Religious Ethics* 13 (1985): 332–59.

———."Bible and Ethics: An Ecclesial and Liturgical Interpretation." *Journal of Religious Ethics* 18 (1990): 129–57.

Gustafson, James M. Introduction to *The Responsible Self*, by H. Richard Niebuhr. New York: Harper and Row, 1963.

Hauerwas, Stanley. "The Moral Authority of Scripture: The Politics and Ethics of Remembering." In *Moral Theology* No. 4, *The Use of Scripture in Moral Theology*, edited by Charles E. Curran and Richard A. McCormick, 242–75. New York: Paulist Press, 1984.

———.*Suffering Presence*. Notre Dame, Ind.: University of Notre Dame Press, 1986.

"It's Over, Debbie." *Journal of the American Medical Association* 259 (8 Jan. 1988): 272.

Johnson, Elizabeth A. *She Who Is: The Mystery of God in Feminist Theological Discourse*. New York: Crossroad, 1994.

Lakoff, George, and Mark Johnson. *Metaphors We Live By*. Chicago: University of Chicago Press, 1980.

MacIntyre, Alasdair. "Theology, Ethics, and the Ethics of Medicine and Health Care." *Journal of Medicine and Philosophy* 4 (1979): 435–43.

May, William F. *The Patient's Ordeal*. Bloomington: Indiana University Press, 1991.

———."The Virtues in a Professional Setting." *Soundings* 67 (1984): 245–66.

McCormick, Richard A. "Theology and Bioethics: Christian

Foundations." In *Theology and Bioethics*, edited by E. Shelp, 95–114. Dordrecht, Netherlands: D. Riedel Publishing Company, 1985.

McGill, Arthur C. *Suffering: A Test of Theological Method*. Philadelphia: Westminster Press, 1968.

Miller, Arthur. *Death of a Salesman*. In *The Portable Arthur Miller*, edited by Harold Clurman, 3–133. New York: Viking Press, 1971.

Niebuhr, Reinhold. *An Interpretation of Christian Ethics*. San Francisco: Harper and Row, 1935.

O'Connor, Flannery. "A Good Man Is Hard to Find." In *The Complete Stories*, 117–33. New York: Farrar, Straus, and Giroux, 1971.

———. *The Habit of Being*. Edited by Sally Fitzgerald. New York: Random House, 1980.

Price, Reynolds. *Kate Vaiden*. New York: Ballantine Books, 1986.

Sölle, Dorothee. *Suffering*. Philadelphia: Fortress Press, 1975.

Updike, John. "From the Journal of a Leper." In *Problems and Other Stories*, 181–96. New York: Alfred A. Knopf, 1979.

Wilder, Thornton. *The Angel That Troubled the Waters*. In *The Angel That Troubled the Waters and Other Plays*, 145–49. New York: Coward-McCann, Inc., 1928.

Wood, Charles M. *The Formation of Christian Understanding*. Valley Forge, Pa.: Trinity Press, 1981.

INDEX

❖